Frontiers in Fracture Management

Frontiers in Fracture Management

edited by

Timothy D. Bunker,
BSc, MCh Orth, FRCS, FRCSEd
Senior Registrar

Christopher L. Colton
FRCS, FRCSEd
Consultant Surgeon

and

John K. Webb
FRCS
Consultant Surgeon

*Department of Fracture and Orthopaedic
Surgery
University Hospital
Queen's Medical Centre
Nottingham*

MARTIN DUNITZ

First published in the United Kingdom in 1989
by Martin Dunitz Ltd, 154 Camden High Street, London NW1 0NE

British Library Cataloguing in Publication Data

Frontiers in fracture management.
1. Man. Bones. Fractures. Therapy
I. Bunker, Timothy D.   II. Colton,
Christopher L.   III. Webb, John K.
617′.15

ISBN 0–948269–37–5

Phototypeset by Latimer Trend & Company Ltd, Plymouth
Origination by Paramount Litho, Essex
Printed in the United Kingdom at the University Press, Cambridge

Contents

Introduction

This book is intended for senior residents and trauma surgeons as an update on controversies at the frontiers of fracture care. The book has been deliberately written as a scientific contribution intended to counteract some of the inertia which has beset much of trauma care over the past three decades. This is not to say that conservative management has been jettisoned. Indeed, with the latest developments in functional bracing, it is being championed; but all the chapters are based on painstaking scientific research by active young trauma surgeons.

The book is roughly divided into two sections, seven chapters on general fracture care and five chapters on specific fracture topics. It is appropriate that the book starts with fracture planning, about which little has previously been written. The next two chapters describe recent advances in the perception of the dynamics of wound infection in fractures and modern techniques of wound cover. Our understanding of fracture healing and bone grafting continues to improve and the next two chapters describe the current state of the art of these basic biological processes. Major advances in our understanding of the physiological effects of polytrauma have occurred in the last decade and consequently our principles in polytrauma management have been radically altered, as explained in Chapter 6. The final chapter on general topics examines the ever-growing problems associated with the epidemic of fractures in the elderly.

The first of the specific topics is on the Herbert differential-pitch bone screw, an entirely new principle in screw design, and its use in scaphoid and osteochondral fractures. Many controversies surround the management of proximal humeral fractures and in Chapter 9 the recent cycle of enthusiasm and despair over their conservative and surgical management is reviewed. Advances in thermoplastic materials have brought about a revolution in bracing methods, which have been pioneered in Sheffield and Manchester, and these are discussed in the next chapter. Locking medullary nailing has expanded the indications of an already valuable operation and its potential is in the middle of a growth spurt which is far from fully developed. The final chapter discusses the renaissance of external fixation brought about by our understanding of frame biomechanics, fracture healing and pin sepsis, which have expanded its indications beyond even the dreams of a decade ago.

Trauma care is for ever evolving, and even if some of the present spectacular frontiers of fracture management eventually become outmoded, it is our intention to inspire the next generation of trauma surgeons to question dogma, to think biologically and to strive for perfection for the traumatized patient.

Timothy D. Bunker,
Christopher L. Colton,
John K. Webb
Nottingham, 1989

Acknowledgments

Figures are reproduced with the kind permission of the following: W B Saunders Company (Figures 2.1, 2.2); C V Mosby Company (Figure 2.4, reproduced from: Burke J F, The effective period of preventative antibiotic action in experimental incisions and dermal lesions, *Surgery* (1961) **50:** 161–8); Professor Robert Schenk (Figures 4.3, 4.4, 4.7, reproduced from: Schenk R, Willeneger H, Morphological findings in primary fracture healing, *Symposia Biologica Molecula* (1967) **8:** 75–86); *Journal of Trauma* (Figures 6.3, 6.4, reproduced from: Baker SP, O'Neill B, Haddon W Jr, The injury severity score: A method for describing patients with multiple injuries and evaluating emergency care (1974) **14:** 187–96); Professor R Salter and the American Academy of Surgeons Instructional Course Lectures (Figure 8.7); *Journal of Bone and Joint Surgery* (Figure 8.9, reproduced from: Bunker TD, Scott TD, MacNamee PB, A multicenter study of the Herbert differential pitch bone screw for scaphoid fractures (1987) **69B:** 631–8, and Figures 8.15 and 8.17, reproduced from: MacNamee PB, Bunker TD, Scott TD, The Herbert differential pitch bone screw for articular and osteochondral fractures (1988) **70B:** 145–6); *Injury* (Figure 8.11, reproduced from: Bunker TD, Newman JH, The Herbert differential pitch bone screw in radial head fractures (1985) **16:** 621) by permission of Butterworth & Co (Publishers) Ltd; Rizzoli Institute, Bologna (Figure 11.7); Charles C Thomas, Publisher, Springfield, Illinois (Figures 12.4, 12.5, 12.6, reproduced from: Green SA, *Complications of External Fixation*, 1981).

Acknowledgments are due for supplying illustrations to the Departments of Medical Illustration, at the Royal Infirmary, Cardiff, for Figures 4.1, 4.2, 4.3, 4.8, and at the University Hospital, Nottingham, for help with illustrations in most chapters, in particular Chapter 1, with special thanks to Yvonne Tennie, medical photographer.

1

Planning in fracture surgery

B. J. Holdsworth, BSc, MB, BS, FRCS

The concept of drawing detailed plans before embarking on an operation is familiar to all orthopaedic surgeons in the field of corrective osteotomy. However, in fracture fixation, this discipline is more often paid lip-service than observed.

An acknowledged master of the planning method, and also of the three-dimensional thinking required, is M. E. Müller of Berne, a founder member of the AO group of Swiss surgeons. His own abilities as a surgical 'conjuror' may have dissuaded other less dexterous operators from acquiring what I believe to be an essential skill. It is, of course, true that there is no surer way to show one's lack of understanding than to draw up a plan which either proves impossible to implement or which seriously underestimates the problem. With regular use of the planning method, such problems become increasingly rare and a clear concept of surgical feasibility emerges. Thus, if a surgical plan is difficult to visualize on paper, inevitably in the operating theatre it will be virtually impossible. As Geoffrey Mast so succinctly expressed it in a talk on the subject, 'It is better to throw your plans in the rubbish bin than your patients on the scrap heap!'[1]

The planning technique should first be applied in simple fractures, where its use may be optional. Once the method is mastered, it can be carried through into more complex situations which are thereby rendered safer, less strenuous for the surgeon and the patient, and often considerably quicker.

Planning materials

The first prerequisite is a series of good radiographs. It may be impossible to obtain perfect anteroposterior and lateral projections of the fracture, but it is always possible to take control radiographs of the opposite limb, and when reversed they give a scale model on which to assemble the fracture fragments. If there is comminution, oblique views of the fracture should also be taken before commencing the operation. In the case of fracture dislocations, it is often possible to achieve a provisional reduction by manipulation, under anaesthesia if necessary. Additional radiographs taken then may give a much clearer idea of what exactly is required.

Certain fractures require more intensive radiographic analysis, for example, tomography in the case of depressed fractures of the tibial plateaux. Even in these cases, most of the fracture fragments may be discerned on good quality plain anteroposterior, lateral and oblique films, which can usually be obtained on arrival and may clarify the need, or otherwise, for tomography. Computer-aided tomography (CAT scanning) is becoming increasingly appropriate, especially in treating acetabular or other pelvic fractures.

It is a common error to accept films of poor quality, taken under duress when the patient first arrives, perhaps multiply injured, in the accident department. In such cases, it is suggested that further films are taken under anaesthesia if necessary, after resuscitation and immediately prior to internal fixation. The slight delay while plans are then drawn is amply repaid in time saved in searching for implants or in operating through an inappropriate incision.

Good quality tracing paper is a bonus, but any strong and slightly transparent material will suffice so long as the radiographs are clearly visible through it when placed on a viewing box. The clear cellophane with paper backing used in many operating theatres for wrapping instruments before sterilization may be close at hand.

A full set of scale templates from the range of internal fixation devices is available from the AO group and is often of great assistance in planning with accuracy (Figure 1.1).[2]

Finally, a selection of coloured pens with fine points helps to differentiate the fragments, although a sharp pencil should be used for the initial tracing.

Drawing the plans

The first step is to trace each fragment of the fracture separately, using the best of the plain radiographs (Figure 1.2a). This entails careful study of the tips of the main fragments in order to avoid missing real or potential 'butterfly' fragments. As a broad generalization, virtually all fractures of a spiral nature have this potential, owing to indirect trauma. The faintest hint of a 'hairline' crack, extending up or down from the main fracture gap and in line with one face of the main fracture, is a warning of possible trouble (see Figure 1.4a). A single lag screw to control this propagating fissure may be all that is required to prevent the embarrassing occurrence of a refracture just above the plate.

Figure 1.1 There are templates available of virtually the whole range of AO implants. These are at the typical magnification of average radiographs (ie, 1.1:1).

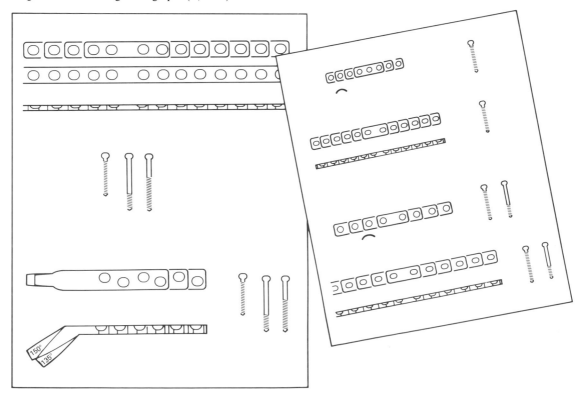

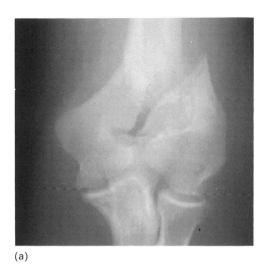

(a)

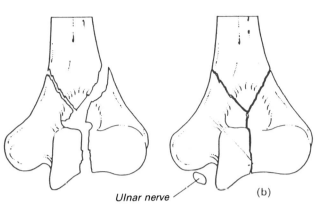

Ulnar nerve

(b)

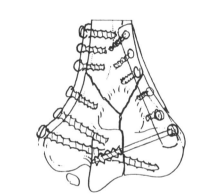

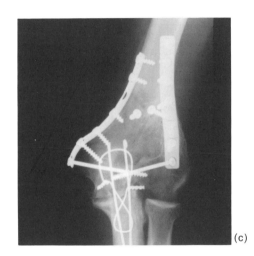

(c)

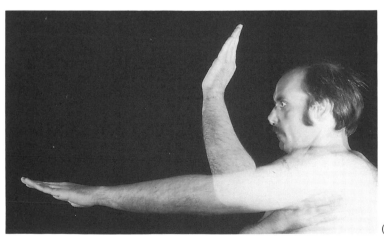

(d)

Figure 1.2 *a* The first stage is to
determine the shape, number and
size of the various fragments.
b The fragments are assembled on
a tracing of the normal side,
reversed. In the unusual event of
severe bilateral fractures,
templates of standard size bones
are also available. *c* If the plan is
followed carefully during the
operation, it should closely
resemble the final radiographs.
d Clinical success is then to be
expected.

(a)

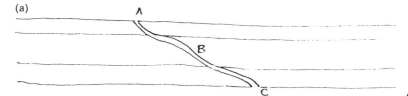

A simple short oblique fracture

(b)

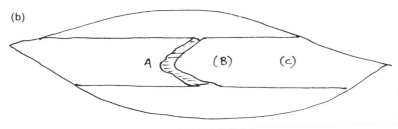

The view of the fracture via a (correctly) gentle dissection may deceive.

(c)

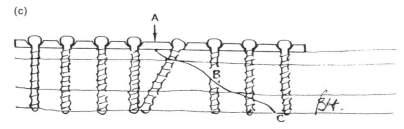

Plate (wrongly) centred at A—note poor hold on the right-hand fragments.

(d)

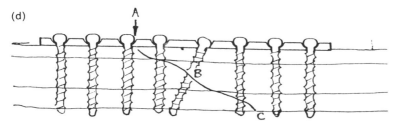

A better postition of the same implants gives a much more stable fixation.

Figure 1.3 This shows how planning may allow a more correct position of implants than is apparently obvious at operation when soft tissues may obscure the view.

While tracing these fragments, it is vital to note the orientation of the principal bone spikes in the plane perpendicular to the drawing. Two drawings at right angles are needed in most cases to allow the development of a clear, three-dimensional image of the fracture (Figure 1.4*b*). If possible, a dry bone or plastic replica should be at hand, on which the fracture lines can be marked. Once the exact number and shape of the various pieces are known, they can be traced on to the reversed outline of the normal limb and assembled in the 'best fit' position (Figure 1.2*b*).

Despite the inevitable minor inaccuracy introduced by differences in rotation of some fragments relative to the plane of the radiograph, a surprisingly true representation of the operative findings is usually achieved.

Having built a clear picture of the fracture, it remains to add the internal fixation device to the drawing (Figure 1.2*b*). Fortunately, assuming the AO style of implants are used, templates are available of the whole range of devices at a magnification of 1.1:1, which closely approximates to that of standard plain radiographs. If the plan is followed accurately, it should closely resemble the final radiograph (Figure 1.2*c*). Clinical success is then to be expected (Figure 1.2*d*).

Choice of implants

It is difficult to give clear guidelines as to exactly how many screws, or how long a plate, are required in each case. In the forearm bones, for example, three screws are usually safest and should be used whenever possible, providing six cortical holds in each of the main fragments (this is not counting the interfragmentary screws). In fixing lower limb fractures, where the spiral is often longer, it is sometimes possible to use a plate with only two screws beyond the limits of the fracture. Some surgeons may feel that this is excessively cautious, but it is advisable not to use shorter plates until considerable experience has been gained.

The pattern of each screw to be used, and which particular screws should be lagged to achieve interfragmentary compression, can be decided in advance and marked on the diagram. Such details, once mastered by the scrub nurse, can save a considerable amount of operating time.

Prediction of stability and need for bone grafting

Planning can help in predicting the likely degree of rigidity of the proposed fixation as well as any probable cortical defects. In certain circumstances, bone grafting of the fixed fracture is definitely required, for example, in severely comminuted tibial fractures or in the few cases of femoral shaft fracture in which plating is used. Again, this is a requirement that can be planned ahead. The donor site is then always accessible and prepared in advance, and no disturbance of the sterile field occurs should a graft become necessary. In tibial fractures, the graft is usually taken before the tourniquet is inflated, thereby avoiding excessive tourniquet times.

Considerations

If this form of careful planning is carried out, the internal fixation itself will become a lot easier as the pattern unfolds. Also, by having studied the 'blueprint', the required instruments or fixation devices will have been laid out.

Most failures of internal fixation are due to technical errors; for example, fixation with plates which are of inadequate length or are wrongly centred, assuming that accurate reduction has been achieved. Many such instances can be avoided if preoperative plans are followed. It is often much clearer to decide on the plan exactly where the plate should be centred than in the restricted view afforded by the wound, unless soft tissue is stripped to such an extent as to endanger the viability of the bone (Figure 1.3).

Examples of planning

The case illustrated in Figure 1.4 is a deceptively simple tibial shaft fracture resulting from a low energy accident. On close inspection, the radiographs revealed a propagating crack which may easily have become a frank 'butterfly' fragment. Such fragments are, indeed, often already separate when the fracture is opened. This potential 'butterfly' fragment was therefore in the plan, as shown in Figure 1.4*b*; the plate was centred over it. The plan was successfully followed and, despite the patient being elderly and suffering from severe Parkinson's disease, he was able to start walking quite soon (Figure 1.4*c* and *d*).

The advantage of planning in determining which implant is required in a particular fracture is illustrated in the two cases on pages 8 and 9.

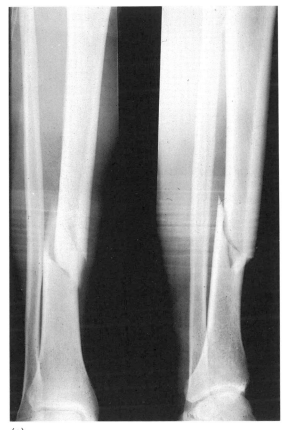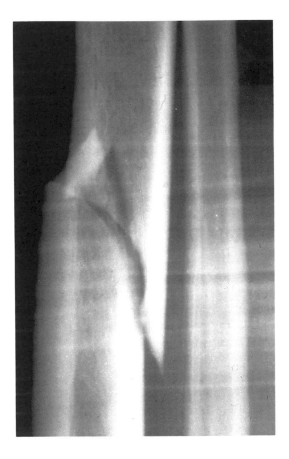

(a)

Figure 1.4 *a* The fracture (AP and lateral radiographs);
the close-up shows a propagating crack.
b The plan, including the butterfly fragment.
c and *d* The operative films; the slightly overlong screws
were accepted.

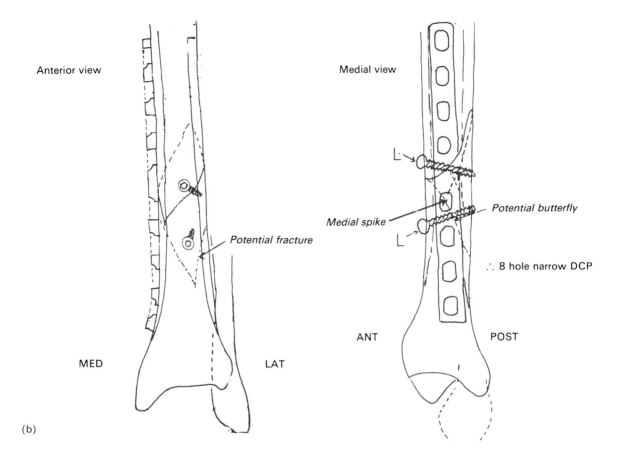

Anterior view

Medial view

Potential fracture

L

L

Medial spike

Potential butterfly

∴ 8 hole narrow DCP

MED

LAT

ANT

POST

(b)

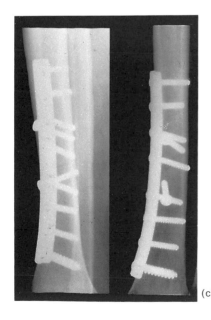

(c)

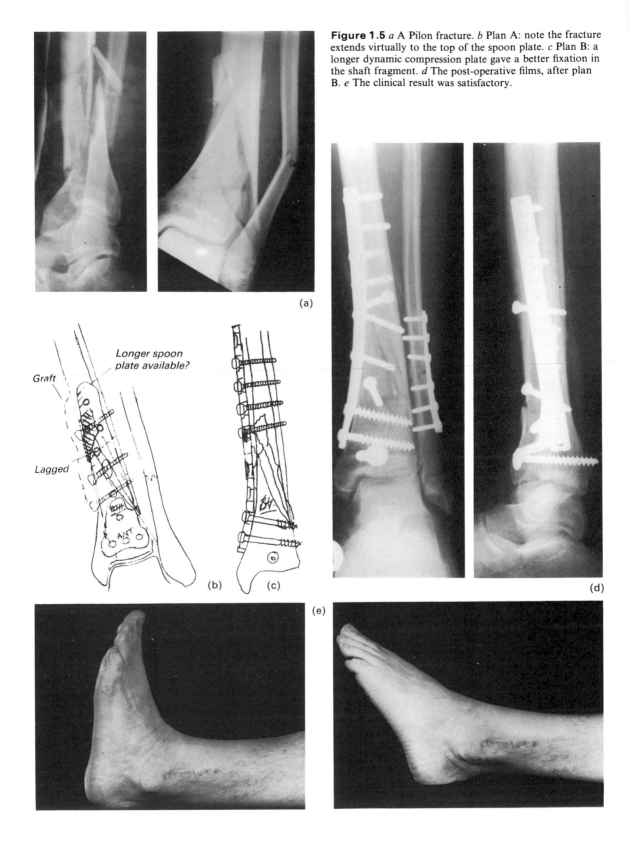

Figure 1.5 *a* A Pilon fracture. *b* Plan A: note the fracture extends virtually to the top of the spoon plate. *c* Plan B: a longer dynamic compression plate gave a better fixation in the shaft fragment. *d* The post-operative films, after plan B. *e* The clinical result was satisfactory.

Longer spoon plate available?

Graft

Lagged

(a)

(b)

(c)

(d)

(e)

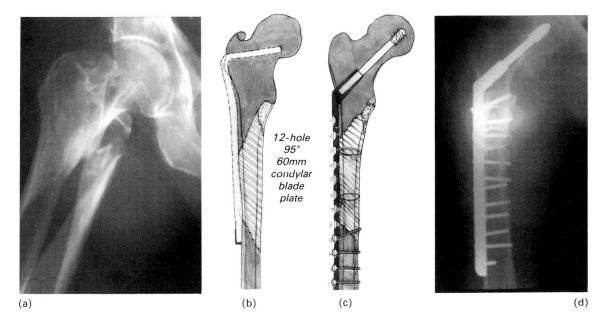

(a) (b) (c) (d)

12-hole
95°
60mm
condylar
blade
plate

Figure 1.6 *a* A long spiral fracture in the proximal
femur. *b* The longest condylar blade plate in theatre
would, after all, have been too short. *c* A 12-hole dynamic
hip screw seemed more promising. *d* This second plan was
successful and the patient rapidly mobilized.

Case 1

A comminuted 'Pilon' fracture of the lower tibia
(Figure 1.5*a*) was at first thought to be suitable for a
'spoon' plate, which in this situation usually gives
good fixation (Figure 1.5*b*). However, as shown on
the plan, this plate would have only just reached the
upper limit of the fracture. Therefore a second plan
was drawn, this time using a contoured dynamic
compression plate (DCP) with additional interfragmentary screws (Figure 1.5*c*). This second plan was
followed with a good result (Figure 1.6*d* and *e*).

Case 2

This was a long, spiral fracture of the upper femur in
an elderly man (Figure 1.6*a*). In recent practice, the
usual implant for this type of fracture is a condylar
blade plate. The longest plate of this type available in
the operating theatre was a twelve-hole, and preoperative planning showed this length to be inadequate
(Figure 1.6*b*). A further plan was drawn, this time
using a twelve-hole dynamic hip screw (DHS; Figure
1.6*c*): the DHS has a longer effective reach than a

DCP for the same number of holes. It is also easier to
insert correctly and more tolerant of any persisting
medial cortical defect. This second plan was followed
successfully and the patient rapidly became mobile
(Figure 1.6*d*).

Plans do not always present the full picture and,
occasionally, despite careful scrutiny of the films,
comminution is worse than anticipated. Figure 1.7*a*
shows an apparently simple displaced fracture of the
medial condyle of the humerus, but with a crack in
the lateral condyle. It was hoped to fix this crack by a
single screw (Figure 1.7*b*). However, in order to gain
access to both condyles, an olecranon osteotomy was
decided upon and, in cutting the bone, the lateral
condyle was displaced. This necessitated an additional small plate, as shown on the postoperative
radiographs (Figure 1.7*c*). The outcome was successful (Figure 1.7*d*).

Some of the most challenging fractures to fix are
the severely comminuted and displaced intercondylar
fractures of the elbow. Figure 1.8*a* shows such a
fracture in a twenty-two-year-old motor-cyclist. The
preoperative plan and the final radiographs are
remarkably similar (Figure 1.8*b*). The clinical result

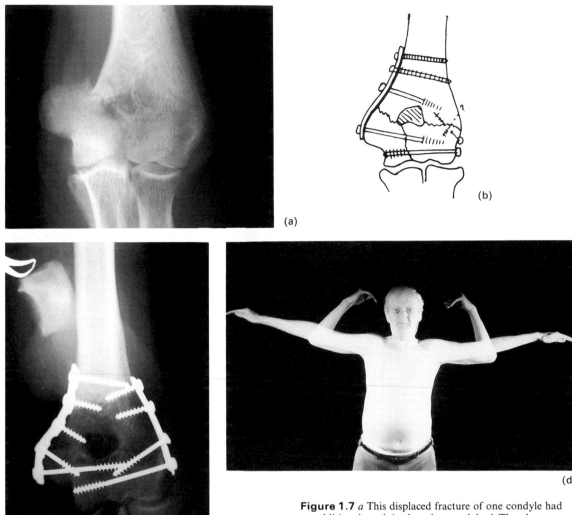

Figure 1.7 *a* This displaced fracture of one condyle had an additional crack in the other condyle. *b* The plan was to fix the crack by a single screw. *c* A second small plate was required when the second condyle displaced during the operation. Note that this did not materially alter the pattern of the fixation.
d The outcome was acceptable.

was excellent, with only a 10 degree loss of flexion and extension (Figure 1.8*c* and *d*).

Figure 1.9*a* and *b* shows a similar fracture. Again, the plan provided an accurate guide during the operation (Figure 1.9*c* and *d*). In both these cases of severe articular fractures, good clinical results were achieved despite apparently excessive internal fixation. Both patients are now back in their heavy manual occupations, with few complaints.

Such complex fractures should never be undertaken without planning, by no means a new concept. In 1940, in an article on intercondylar fractures, Van Gorder said, 'Too much emphasis cannot be placed upon this matter of preliminary preparation . . . without it the operation should not be undertaken'.[3]

The final case illustrates many of the benefits of planning: a twenty-three-year-old woman was travelling with her left elbow out of the car window when,

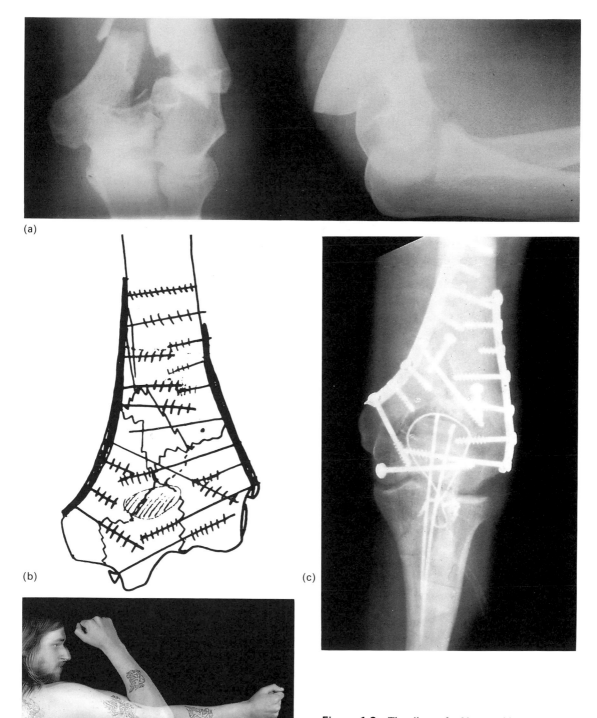

(a)

(b)

(c)

(d)

Figure 1.8 *a* The elbow of a 22-year-old motor-cyclist.
b The plan. Again note the olecranon fossa is preserved.
c The operative films closely match the plan. *d* Stable
fixation allowed early active movement leading to this
result at eighteen months.

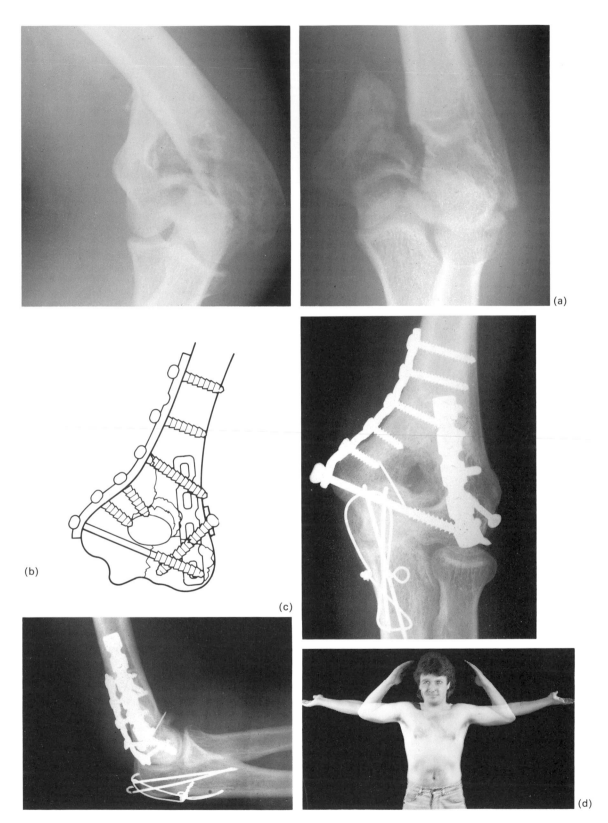

Figure 1.9 *a* A severe distal humeral fracture. *b* The plan. Care has been taken to avoid blocking the olecranon fossa. *c* The fixation achieved.*d* The patient was back working as an underground miner at four months.

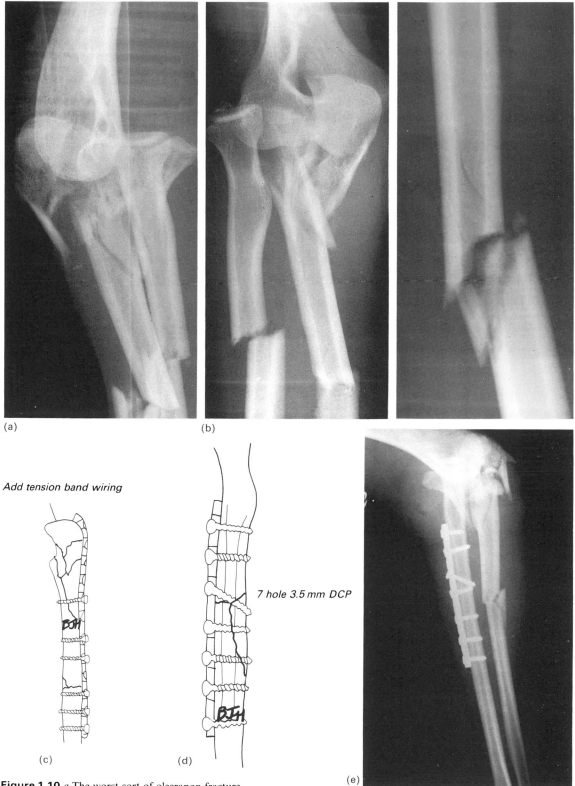

(a)

(b)

Add tension band wiring

BJH

(c)

7 hole 3.5 mm DCP

BJH

(d)

(e)

Figure 1.10 *a* The worst sort of olecranon fracture.
b The ipsi-lateral forearm; note the radial and ulnar shaft
fractures. *c* A basic plan for the comminuted ulna
suggested the longest 3.5 DCP would just suffice. *d* The
radial fracture was simple to plan. *e* The first step was to
fix the radius. (*continued*)

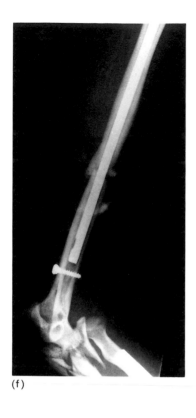

(f)

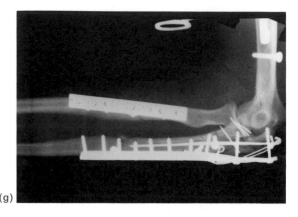

(g)

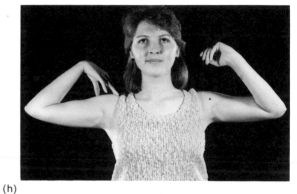

(h)

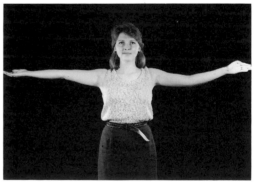

Figure 1.10 *continued f* Second, the humerus was nailed, via the elbow fracture. *g* The jigsaw of the ulnar fracture was then reassembled. Note how closely the length of the plate corresponds to the plan. This was crucial, otherwise fixation of the ulnar shaft would have been lost. *h* The patient required one further procedure on the humerus. This is her function at nine months.

in a collision with another vehicle, she sustained a 'baby-car' fracture (Figure 1.10*a*). In addition to a frightfully smashed proximal ulna, she sustained a fracture of the left humeral shaft with a 'butterfly' fragment, as well as fractures in the shafts of the left radius and ulna with slight comminution (Figure 1.10*b*). The hand was well perfused, with intact sensation.

Preoperative planning suggested that both ulnar fractures could be controlled adequately by the longest 3.5 mm DCP that was readily available (Figure 1.10*c*), and the radial shaft by a shorter plate (Figure 1.10*d*). It would have been possible to plate the humerus, but not without a very extensive exposure and with potential danger to the radial nerve.

Such a combined internal fixation was predicted to take many hours. It was thought best to use a tourniquet during both the elbow fixation and the radial plating, in order safely to visualize the neurovascular structures. The scheme entailed plating of the radial fracture via an anterior 'Henry' approach, thus restoring the length of the forearm; the latter was under a tourniquet (Figure 1.10e).

The tourniquet was released and the patient remained prone for the rest of the operation. The humeral fracture was fixed via the olecranon fracture, using a narrow nail inserted through the olecranon fossa. A transverse screw supported the nail (Figure 1.10f).

The tourniquet was then reapplied, and the painstaking task of reassembling the ulna was carried out (Figure 1.10g). Surprisingly, perhaps, the fixation of the elbow, once tension band reinforcement was added, proved quite secure and the patient was treated in a continuous passive motion machine for several weeks. For most of this time she was at home, and regained an excellent range of elbow movement. However, the humeral fracture was problematic and went on to delayed union requiring later removal of the nail, plating and grafting. Figure 1.10h shows the patient's function after the second procedure.

Postoperative care

It must be realized that the results shown in these examples were obtained only after meticulous postoperative supervision. The aim of this method of fixation is to enable very early restoration of movement, with the intention of avoiding the problems of 'fracture disease'. It is imperative that the patients realize their role in this respect and cooperate accordingly. It may be best to avoid internal fixation in patients who show no signs of such cooperation.

In the case of the elbow joint, passive stretching is, in general, forbidden. The use of a passive motion machine seems an exception, possibly because in most cases it becomes comfortable very rapidly, and hence muscle tone is reduced. Early active movements are started in all cases when suction drains are removed, usually forty-eight hours after the operation. The limb is elevated in a well padded splint.

The use of ancillary external splintage, once soft tissue healing has occurred, is a point of controversy. Nevertheless, the use of a well constructed cast brace, which allows joint motion while reducing the amplitude of cyclical stress on the internal fixation, has something to commend it. However, few of the cases examined here had, in fact, any external support.

Full weight-bearing is not allowed until it is thought that bony union has at least commenced. This can be difficult to judge if fixation has been successful in obliterating the fracture lines and in maintaining rigidity, which prevents callus. As a rule of thumb we have accepted that, by six to eight weeks in most cases, the fracture/metal complex is strong enough to allow unprotected use.

Conclusion

Despite the benefits of formal planning, there are disadvantages, which may be summarized as follows:

1. Advance planning is time-consuming (about half an hour in difficult cases).

2. Plans require the ability to trace carefully and to interpret the radiographs accurately in three dimensions. This, in some fractures, can be very difficult.

3. They provide a sure way of demonstrating the surgeon's lack of understanding of either the fracture or the principles of internal fixation.

4. What seems ideal on paper may prove impossible to carry through at operation, although this is quite rare. Sometimes slight adjustments are required, as seen in our case studies, but plans are always versatile.

The advantages of planning are great, and may be summarized as follows:

1. Planning helps the surgeon to clarify his thoughts, by sharpening his three-dimensional perception of radiographic appearances and reducing frequency of 'getting out of one's depth'.

2. It helps to avoid implants which are inappropriate in size, type or position.

3. It helps to determine the optimal surgical approach.

4. It assists the theatre nurse in preparing the correct instruments.

5. Operating time is reduced.

6. Planning may thus reduce traffic in and out of the theatre and so minimize turbulence and possible wound contamination.

7. The difficulty of devising a suitable plan may act as a warning not to embark on an impossible internal fixation.

2

The prevention of infection in open fractures

Peter Worlock, MB, BS, DM,
FRCS (Edin), FRCS (Eng)

Open fractures still present a major therapeutic challenge to the orthopaedic surgeon. This is primarily because of infection, which is the main cause of amputation, non-union and poor functional and cosmetic results in these patients. The prevention of infection is, therefore, the main priority in the treatment of open fractures.

Historical background

The management of contaminated wounds has taxed the skill of surgeons through the ages. The history of the management of such injuries is mainly the history of military surgery. The descriptions of wound treatment in the Edwin Smith Surgical Papyrus, which dates from 1600–1500 BC, indicates that Egyptian physicians were dressing wounds with grease, honey and lint. In biblical times, other methods of antisepsis were in vogue, as the description of the Good Samaritan reveals: '. . . and bound his wounds, pouring in oil and wine' (Luke **10**:33,34).

There is little written evidence extant about the practices of mediaeval surgeons. However, a fourteenth-century French surgeon, Guy de Chauliac, advocated the enlargement of the wound to provide drainage, the removal of foreign bodies and the use of brandy in dressings.[1] An English surgeon, John Arderne of Newark, who practised at the same time, wrote of the necessity of keeping wounds clean so that they would heal without suppuration.[2] He also advised that wounds should be dressed infrequently and allowed to heal from the bottom upwards.

Yet the teachings of these men remained largely unknown. Ambroise Paré (Figure 2.1) recorded that

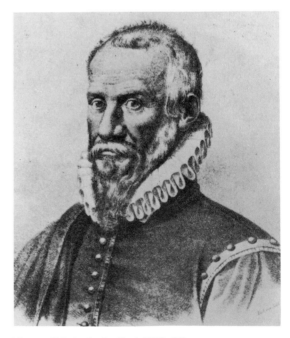

Figure 2.1 Ambroise Paré (1510–90).

gunshot wounds were usually treated at that time by cautery with boiling oil.[3] After his experiences as a military surgeon, Paré recommended enlarging wounds and removing all foreign material before applying a salve to the wound. For open fractures, Paré wrote of the need to leave the wound open and splint the fracture.

By the first half of the nineteenth century fractures with open wounds were regarded as one of the most fatal forms of injury and immediate amputation was often advised.[4] Lister first described the use of carbolic acid as an antiseptic in the treatment of open fractures in 1867.[5] However, there was considerable resistance to his treatments and it took some twenty years for Lister's methods to become widely established. Thereafter, the antiseptic school reigned supreme until the First World War. The value of wound debridement was not accepted, despite the experimental work of Friedrich, who showed that if wound excision was performed within four to six hours of contamination, infection was usually prevented.[6]

During the early months of the First World War, the high infection rate after gunshot wounds forced military surgeons to add wound debridement to their management regimes. As Sir Robert Jones (Figure 2.2) recorded, 'No surgeon had any knowledge of the appalling sepsis which supervened in wounded men who had lain in the mud of Flanders. The dry, clean sun of South Africa and the clean bullet wound had given us all a false impression of the nature of military surgery.'[7] Both British and French army surgeons adopted the practice of thorough wound debridement (thereby removing necrotic tissue and foreign bodies) and then irrigating the wound with hypochlorite solution.

At the start of the First World War, the mortality rate after open fracture of the femur approached 80 per cent. Sir Robert Jones introduced the use of the Thomas splint to stabilize such fractures and the mortality rate fell to 20 per cent. This concept in splintage was taken further by Trueta during the Spanish Civil War.[8] Trueta's methods were based on those of Winnett Orr[9] and consisted of an extensive debridement of the wound, excising all necrotic tissue, and then leaving the wound open. The limb was then immobilized in a plaster of Paris cast, to include the joint above and below the fracture; this cast was retained as long as possible. Trueta reported only six deaths among 1073 patients with open fractures treated in this way. The osteitis rate was 7.6 per cent and a good functional result was seen in over 90 per cent of patients.

During the Second World War, the principles of treatment of open fractures by adequate wound debridement and splintage of the fracture were firmly established. The debate over whether wound closure should be primary or secondary was settled in favour of the latter. This policy of rapid evacuation, wound excision and delayed closure was adopted in both the Korean and Vietnam conflicts, and remains the standard practice for war wounds today. During the Vietnam War, Heaton et al[10] reported infection rates as low as 2.6 per cent after open fractures treated in this way.

Dynamics of wound infection

An understanding of the dynamics of infection in both bone and soft tissue is necessary if infection after open fracture is to be prevented. Most open fractures will be significantly contaminated with bacteria by the time the patient reaches hospital. The work of both Gustilo and Anderson[11] and of Patzakis and Ivler[12] confirms that between 60 and 70 per cent of such

Figure 2.2 Sir Robert Jones.

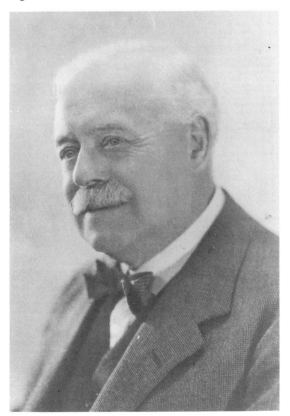

patients will have positive wound cultures before treatment begins.

The size of bacterial inoculum is also of importance in the development of infection. Using quantitative microbiological assessments of traumatic wounds of the hand and forearm, Cooney et al found that sepsis was unlikely to occur with fewer than 10^5 organisms per gram of tissue.[13] The smaller study of Marshall et al confirms that the critical inoculum for the development of infection in man is 10^5 organisms per gram of tissue.[14]

The time between injury and surgical treatment is another important factor, as bacterial proliferation is time-dependent. Robson et al[15] assessed the effect of delay between wounding and treatment on the bacterial colony count in the wound (Table 2.1). There was an average delay of over five hours in those wounds with over 10^5 organisms per gram of tissue. The work of Robson et al confirms the earlier observations of Edlich et al[16] and Friedrich's original experiments in 1898.[6] The time factor is important because once the colony count rises above 10^5 organisms per gram of tissue, wound infection is likely.[13,14,16]

In experimental infections of skin wounds there is a 'decisive period' in the first four hours after inoculation, during which the eventual outcome is determined. If host defences are inhibited by local ischaemia or shock, the size and extent of the local infection is increased.[17] This 'enhancement' is maximal when the enhancing agent is used in the first four hours after inoculation. It effectively disappears by four to five hours after inoculation. If the wound is subjected to such enhancing agents during the decisive period, the critical bacterial inoculum necessary for the development of infection may be reduced.[17]

This early work of Miles et al[17] has been subsequently confirmed.[18,19] It appears that, during the first few hours after inoculation, there is extensive destruction of the primary lodgement of bacteria by the local defences. These defence mechanisms cease to operate after this period and the subsequent course of the local infection is determined by the number of bacteria surviving this early decisive period.

Although the effect of trauma on host defence mechanisms has not been systematically studied, it is likely that these mechanisms are impaired in open fractures because of the presence of oedema, non-viable tissue and ischaemia.[20] It has been shown experimentally that trauma and shock will depress phagocytosis by macrophages and polymorphonuclear leucocytes.[21] Although these changes are normally of short duration and are followed by a 'rebound' effect, initially they may permit bacteria to gain a lodgement at the wound site. Tissue necrosis, ischaemia, haemorrhage and the presence of debris will also decrease the number of bacteria necessary to cause infection.[22]

Classification of open fractures

Before the principles of open fracture management are discussed, it is useful to classify the injury. The severity of the injury to the bone and surrounding soft tissue is important as it will often determine the outcome. A readily useable classification depending on the mechanism of injury, soft tissue damage and the degree of skeletal involvement has been proposed by Gustilo (Table 2.2).[23]

Using these criteria, Gustilo and colleagues[24] reported an overall infection rate of 4.7 per cent in 727 open fractures treated between 1969 and 1979. There were no infections among the 326 Type I open fractures, while the infection rate was 1.8 per cent for Type II injuries (four cases out of 221 fractures). However, thirty of the 180 Type III fractures became infected—an infection rate of 16.7 per cent. Gustilo et al[24] have reviewed their most recent experience with Type III open fractures and recommend that such injuries should be reclassified into three sub-groups (Table 2.3). The practical value of such a classification is that it allows the surgeon to assess the risks and benefits to the patient, when selecting the appropriate method of treatment.

Open fracture management

The aim of the primary treatment of all open fractures is to provide the optimum biological environment for the prevention of infection. There are five principles which should be applied to the management of every open fracture. These are:

1. Prevention of further bacterial contamination

Table 2.1 The relationship between time from injury and bacterial counts in traumatic wounds in man[15]

Mean time after injury (hours)	Bacteria/gram of tissue
2.2	$< 10^2$
3.0	10^2–10^5
5.17	$> 10^5$

Table 2.2 Classification of open fractures[23]

Fracture grade	Type of injury
Type I	Clean puncture wound < 1 cm Minimal muscle contusion No crushing injury Simple fracture without comminution
Type II	Laceration > 1 cm without extensive soft tissue damage, flaps or avulsions Minimal to moderate crushing injury Simple fracture without comminution
Type III	Extensive soft tissue damage including skin, muscle and neuro-vascular structures High energy injury with severe crushing component Comminuted fracture component (includes all segmental fractures, all fractures with bone loss, gunshot wounds, traumatic amputations and farm injuries with soil contamination)

Table 2.3 Classification of Type III open fractures[24]

Fracture grade	Type of injury
Type IIIA	Adequate soft tissue coverage of the bone despite extensive soft tissue laceration or flaps Infection rate 4% Amputation rate 0%
Type IIIB	Extensive soft tissue injury with periosteal stripping and bone exposure Major wound contamination Infection rate 52% Amputation rate 16%
Type IIIC	Open fracture associated with an arterial injury requiring repair Infection rate 42% Amputation rate 42%

2. Prevention of bacterial growth

3. Wound debridement

4. Stabilization of the fracture

5. Delayed wound closure.

These five basic principles will now be considered in some detail.

Prevention of further contamination

All open fracture wounds should be considered as contaminated on arrival in hospital. Wound cultures, both aerobic and anaerobic, should be taken before antibiotics are given or the wound debrided. If an organism is isolated, it is likely to be the infecting organism should infection subsequently develop.[25] Identification of bacteria will also aid rational antibiotic policy.

After wound culture swabs have been taken, the wound should be covered by a sterile dressing soaked in an appropriate antiseptic solution, such as povidone-iodine. This dressing is left undisturbed until definitive wound care is performed in the operating theatre. At the Nottingham University Hospital, UK, a Polaroid camera is always available in the Accident Unit. Every open fracture is photographed immediately before being covered with a sterile dressing (Figure 2.3). This visual evidence removes the temptation for all members of the surgical team to remove the dressing and inspect the wound. The effectiveness of such a regime has been demonstrated by Tscherne et al,[26] who reported an infection rate of 4.3 per cent in wounds covered immediately with a sterile dressing. The infection rate was 18.2 per cent in those wounds left exposed until surgery.

Prevention of bacterial growth

There are two major factors that will influence the exponential rise of bacterial numbers in the wound. The first is the delay between injury and definitive wound surgery. The work of Robson et al suggests that the critical inoculum of 10^5 organisms per gram of tissue will be reached in five to six hours in most wounds.[15] This time factor is influenced by the degree of contamination, as the critical bacterial inoculum will be reached far sooner in a heavily contaminated wound. It should be remembered that the presence of shock, tissue necrosis and haematoma will reduce the size of the critical bacterial inoculum necessary for the development of infection.[17,22]

Ideally, all open fractures should be regarded as surgical emergencies and should be definitively treated within six hours of injury. However, there is little objective evidence to support this, although Tscherne et al have reported lower infection rates in patients who were rapidly transferred from the site of accident to the operating room.[26] It has also been suggested that if an open fracture is left untreated for over eight hours, it is converted from a contaminated wound into an infected wound.[23]

The second major factor in the prevention of bacterial growth is the use of antibiotics. The work of Burke,[18] using experimental skin wounds in guinea pigs, showed that antibiotics should be present in the tissues in adequate concentrations *before* inoculation with bacteria if the maximum effect is to be gained

(Figure 2.4). In Burke's animals, the effect of antibiotics became progressively less as their administration was delayed later after inoculation. If the first dose of antibiotic was not given until three or more hours after inoculation, antibiotics had no effect on the outcome. This study forms the base for the rational use of prophylactic antibiotics in elective surgery.

However, recent work from Nottingham[27] suggests that Burke's observations, on the progressive diminution of antibiotic effect, do not apply to experimental bone infections. An experimental model of post-traumatic osteitis was developed using a fracture of the tibia in rabbits, stabilized with an intramedullary rod. The maximum reduction in the rate of osteitis was seen when antibiotics were given before inoculation with bacteria, but antibiotics still produced a reduction in the infection rate if the first dose was delayed until after inoculation. This effect persisted for four hours after inoculation (Table 2.4). In contrast to Burke's observations,[18] there was no progressive reduction in the effect of antibiotics with increasing delay in administering the first dose.

Clinical evidence for the routine use of antibiotics remains conflicting. Some workers report that antibiotics have no effect in preventing infection after open fractures[28-30] and believe that the complications of antibiotic therapy outweigh the possible advantages.[28] The North American experience is in favour of the use of antibiotics.[11,24,25] The one large, prospective, controlled trial carried out by Patzakis and colleagues demonstrated a significant reduction in infection rates when high dose cephalosporins were used.[25]

Appropriate antibiotics should be routinely used in the management of open fractures. They should be given as soon as possible after injury, but after wound cultures have been taken. The choice of antibiotic is dictated by the potential bacterial contamination. Although *Staphylococcus aureus* is the main infecting organism in open fractures,[11,25] there has been a recent increase in the number of Gram-negative infections after Type III open fractures.[24]

A first-generation cephalosporin remains suitable for Type I and Type II open fractures. Cephalosporins are preferable to the synthetic penicillins because of their broader spectrum of activity. Antibiotics should be given intravenously, at maximum dosage. A combination of a first-generation cephalosporin and an aminoglycoside or a third-generation cephalosporin alone is currently recommended for Type III open fractures.[24] If anaerobic contamination is suspected, metronidazole should be added to the antibiotic regime. The choice of antibiotic can be modified according to the results of the initial wound cultures.

The ideal duration of therapy remains to be clarified, but three days' treatment is now advised for uncomplicated injuries.[20,24] Longer courses may lead

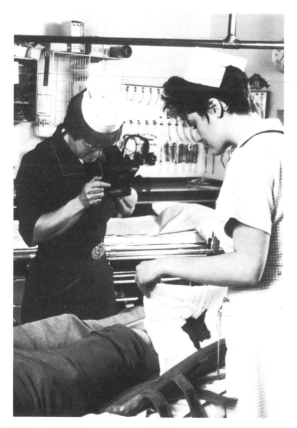

Figure 2.3 The open wound is photographed with a Polaroid camera and then covered with a sterile dressing, soaked in povidone-iodine.

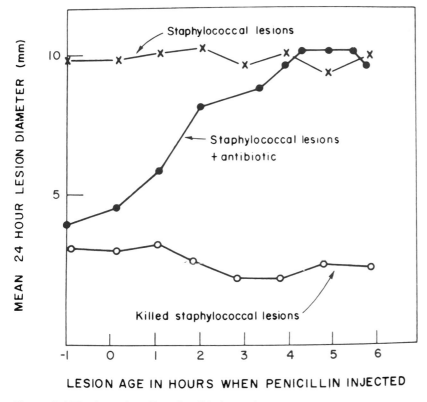

Figure 2.4 The decreasing effect of antibiotics on the extent of experimental skin infections with increasing delay in giving antibiotic after bacterial inoculation.

Table 2.4 The osteitis rate in relation to the delay in starting antibiotic therapy[27]

Group	No of rabbits in group	No of rabbits infected
No antibiotic	11	10
Antibiotic 1 hour pre-inoculation	10	3
Antibiotic 1 hour post-inoculation	11	6
Antibiotic 2 hours post-inoculation	10	5
Antibiotic 3 hours post-inoculation	10	5
Antibiotic 4 hours post-inoculation	10	5
	62 rabbits	

to the appearance of resistant organisms. Appropriate antibiotics should be continued in high dosage if infection supervenes, as an adjunct to the necessary surgical treatment.

It should be clearly understood that antibiotics are not truly prophylactic when used in the management of open fractures. Such wounds are already contaminated with bacteria at the time of antibiotic administration. The antibiotics are, therefore, being used therapeutically.

Wound debridement

Formal wound exploration and debridement in an operating theatre, with the patient adequately anaesthetized, are necessary in all open fractures. The use of a tourniquet should be avoided: inflation of a tourniquet may cause further ischaemic damage to an already compromised limb. Moreover, the determination of tissue viability is made on the basis of colour and bleeding, both of which are modified by the use of a tourniquet. The tourniquet may, however, be applied *uninflated* to the limb and thereafter inflated if absolutely necessary, for brief periods only.

The first stage of debridement is a thorough mechanical cleaning of the wound, using an antiseptic washing agent such as cetrimide. Any major foreign material should be removed at this stage. The wound should then be irrigated with large volumes of normal saline. A minimum of 3 litres is recommended for all wounds[20] and this should be increased to 10–14 litres in extensive wounds.[11,20] Although jet lavage has been described, the simplest method is to use a gravity feed via a standard intravenous giving set (Figure 2.5). The sterile tip of the tube is used as a probe to explore all recesses of the wound and to wash out foreign and

particulate matter.[31] There is no evidence to support the addition of antibiotics to the irrigating solution.

The second stage of debridement is a careful and meticulous exploration of the wound, with excision of all tissue that is dead or of doubtful viability. The open wound should be extended to allow adequate exploration and any crushed or avascular skin and subcutaneous fat must be excised. The deep fascia is opened widely and in the forearm and lower leg a subcutaneous fasciotomy performed. If a compartment syndrome is confirmed by the finding of raised intra-compartmental pressure, formal fasciotomies of the affected compartments should be carried out.

Muscle should be freely excised until the cut edges are pink and bleeding. Vascularized muscle will contract when pinched and this is a reliable sign of viability. All detached small pieces of bone should be removed. The decision as to whether to remove larger devitalized pieces of bone is difficult. Although a major fragment may add to the stability of the fracture, it also represents a potential sequestrum. If the wound is heavily contaminated, such large detached fragments should be removed and the bone loss accepted. The resulting bony defect can be managed by cancellous bone grafting when the soft tissues have healed and the danger of infection has receded.

Throughout this time-consuming stage of wound debridement, the surgeon must take great care not to cause further damage to the tissues. Any additional incisions must be sited carefully to avoid devitalizing adjacent structures. Soft tissue dissection should be kept to a minimum and the tissues handled with care to prevent further interference with the blood supply.

Figure 2.5 Wound irrigation with a standard intravenous giving set. The sterile tip can be used to wash out the recesses of the wound thoroughly.

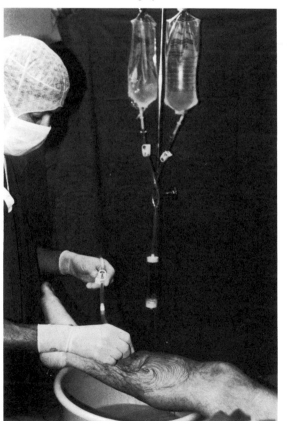

Stabilization of the fracture

Although most surgeons agree that stabilization of an open fracture is important, there is considerable debate as to the degree needed. The controversy is particularly marked over the role of primary internal fixation of open fractures. Traditionally, primary internal fixation has been avoided in the management of open fractures.[11,32] However, various workers have recently advocated the use of internal fixation in open fractures, on the basis that stabilization of the fracture will help prevent the development of sepsis.[29,33,34]

There is no doubt that stability of the fracture is an important factor in the treatment of post-traumatic osteitis. Burri[35] and Weber and Cech,[36] in their extensive clinical reviews, stress that the most important factors in the management of an infected non-union are the resection of all necrotic bone and the stabilization of the fracture by either internal or external fixation.

The hypothesis that stability will favourably affect the outcome in established post-traumatic osteitis has been studied experimentally by Rittmann and Perren.[37] These workers performed tibial osteotomies in sheep and fixed these with plates of varying rigidity, giving three grades of stability. An inoculum of *Staphylococcus aureus* in high concentrations was injected into the wound until infection ensued. Rittmann and Perren concluded that rigid fixation of the osteotomy offered favourable conditions for bone healing, and that the stabilizing effect of implants outweighed the possible disadvantages of a foreign body effect. Although this study supported the concept that stability is of value in treating established osteitis, it threw no light on the question of whether stabilization of a contaminated open fracture would help prevent the development of infection.

Friedrich and Klaue[38] reported that stable fixation of an experimental contaminated fracture in rabbits abolished infection when assessed using clinical criteria. However, they observed radiological and histological signs of infection in animals treated by both stable and unstable fixation. This study is unsatisfactory, as, if stable fixation is of benefit there should be evidence of a diminished osteitis rate with stable fixation, when assessed by strict radiological and histological criteria.

The hypothesis that rigid fixation of a contaminated open fracture reduces its susceptibility to infection has been investigated recently in Nottingham.[39] The tibiae of male New Zealand white rabbits were fractured and then fixed with either a dynamic compression plate ('stable group') or a loose-fitting intramedullary rod ('unstable group'). The fracture site was inoculated with a standard inoculum of *Staphylococcus aureus*. The incidence and progression of osteitis was studied by clinical, radiological, microbiological and histological methods. A strict definition of osteitis was used and there was a statistically significant reduction in the osteitis rate in the stable group (Table 2.5 and Figure 2.6).

Thus, it seems clear that, experimentally, stabilization is of benefit in preventing infection after open fractures, although the mechanism of this remains unclear. Infection in bone depends on an interaction between bacteria and host. Considerable attention has been directed historically to the nature and control of bacteria, with little attention given to the tissues inoculated. Yet Selye[40] reported that Pasteur said on his deathbed, 'The germ is nothing, it is the terrain in which it grows which is everything.'

Khan and Pritzker[41] have stated that three conditions are necessary for the development of osteitis. These are:

1. The presence of bacteria

2. Factors favouring localization of the bacteria

3. Factors favouring bacterial proliferation.

Anatomical reduction and stabilization of a fracture will reduce tissue dead space and decrease the chance of haematoma formation. Conversely, instability at the fracture site will cause local necrosis of the surrounding soft tissues and promote exudate formation, both of which will favour bacterial localization and proliferation.[34,41]

Stability is beneficial to revascularization: Rhinelander et al[42] and Ganz et al[43] have confirmed that blood vessels can be seen crossing an experimental osteotomy within a few days of operation, providing that stability is maintained. However, this revascularization of the fracture site occurs days after injury, and it seems likely that the first few hours after inoculation are critical in determining the outcome.[17,18] Chapman has suggested that stable fixation of a fracture leads to improved tissue perfusion in the adjacent area.[34] This would bring cellular and humeral defences into contact with bacteria. This is an attractive theory, but, as yet, there is little evidence to support it.

Clinically, there are three main methods available for the stabilization of open fractures:

1. External splintage by plaster cast or traction

2. External fixation

3. Internal fixation.

The traditional plaster cast and skeletal traction still allow considerable movement at the fracture site. This is important in promoting healing by external callus formation. However, such motion is not ideal for the prevention of infection and the use of plaster casts or skeletal traction should be reserved for

Table 2.5 Osteitis rate in relation to fracture stability[39]

Group	No of rabbits in group	No of rabbits infected*
Stable (dynamic compression plate)	20	7
Unstable (loose intramedullary rod)	21	15
	41 rabbits	

*$x^2 = 5.47$, DF=1, $p < 0.02$

uncomplicated, stable Type I fractures only. External splintage should not be used in the management of multiple injuries and open intra-articular fractures. Cast and traction techniques must be functionally based, according to the principles of Sarmiento and Latta.[44] The aim of treatment is early weight-bearing using functional braces; muscle wasting and joint stiffness are prevented by isometric muscle exercises and early, active movement.

Type II and Type III open fractures should be stabilized as rigidly as possible with internal or external fixation. External fixation is not as stable as compression plating, but allows excellent access to the wound. The main indications for external fixation are Type III open fractures of the tibia (Figure 2.7) and open fractures of the pelvis. The major problem of pin-tract sepsis can be reduced by a careful insertion technique.[45] Skin necrosis is prevented by adequate

Figure 2.6 Radiographs of rabbit tibiae, obtained 12 weeks after fracture and inoculation with *Staphylococcus aureus*. *a* This stable fracture (fixed with a dynamic compression plate) has healed uneventfully with the radiological appearance of primary bone union. *b* This unstable fracture (fixed with a loose-fitting intramedullary rod) shows obvious signs of infection: periosteal new bone, involucrum formation and osteolysis around the implant.

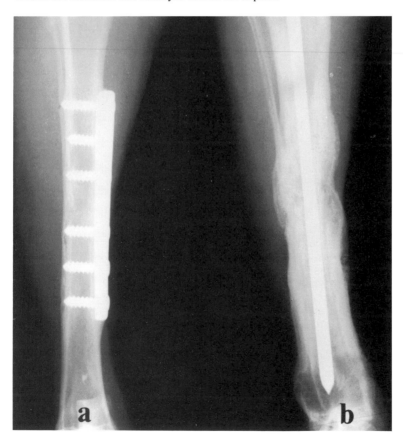

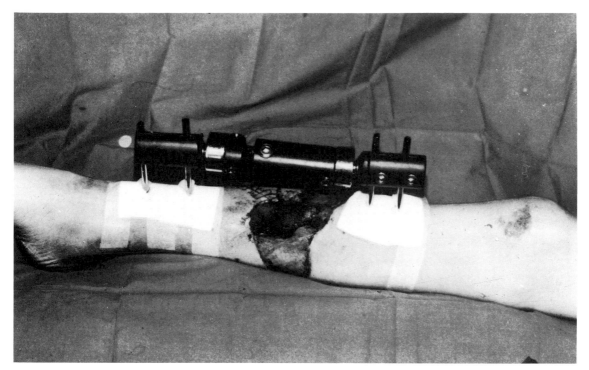

Figure 2.7 The external fixator is the ideal method for stabilizing Type III open fractures of the tibia.

incisions for pin insertion and heat necrosis of bone is avoided by the pre-drilling of bone. Motion at the pin/skin interface can be reduced by the use of bulky, antiseptic-soaked dressings. The use of pins which transfix muscle should be avoided as these are associated with a very high incidence of pin-tract sepsis.[46,47] External fixation of the femur and humerus should be avoided, if possible, because of the inevitable transfixion of the muscles surrounding these bones. The good muscle coverage of the humerus and femur makes these bones much more suitable for stabilization by internal fixation, even in Type III injuries.

The role of primary internal fixation of open fractures remains controversial. This is because of the supposedly higher infection rate after such operations. There are few studies comparing internal fixation with external splintage in the management of open fractures, and all are in the older literature.[48–50] Although all three of these papers reported higher

rates of infection and non-union in the internal fixation groups (see Table 2.6), the techniques used were considerably less refined than those employed today.

Recent work, from major accident units in North America and Europe, suggests that open fractures can be treated by early internal fixation and excellent results obtained (Table 2.7). Although the early infection rate appears high at 7.5 per cent overall, this should be compared with an infection rate of 4.7 per cent overall in a large series of open fractures treated without internal fixation.[24] In all these reports, [24,29,51–54] the infection rate was highest in Type III injuries: these fractures are at an increased risk of infection because of the severity of the injury. La Duca et al[55] reported that the use of primary internal fixation to stabilize these severe injuries allowed improved wound management and contributed to the low infection rate of 4 per cent seen in their patients.

It should also be noted that even if early infection supervenes after primary internal fixation, it is nearly

Table 2.6 Internal fixation versus external splintage in open fractures

| | Internal fixation | | External splintage | |
	Infection	Non-union	Infection	Non-union
Wade and Campbell[48]	14%	27%	3%	9%
Claffey[49]	35%	17%	0%	0%
Gallinaro, Crova and Denicolai[50]	17%	11%	3%	9%

always possible to eradicate it. The stabilizing effect of an implant has a positively beneficial effect on such patients.[35-37] There were only two cases of chronic osteitis out of the 505 open fractures treated in the five studies reported in Table 2.7—an overall rate of 0.4 per cent.[29,51-54]

Primary internal fixation of open fractures remains a difficult and demanding technique. Although doubt was cast on the relationship between metal and bone in the development of infection by Hicks,[56] recent work has demonstrated that the presence of foreign materials (including stainless steel and polymethylmethacrylate) will reduce the critical number of bacteria necessary to cause infection.[57-59] Primary internal fixation of open fractures should be performed only by those surgeons experienced in the technique, working in a unit with the necessary equipment and back-up facilities. Surgery should be carefully planned and meticulously performed. All surgical incisions should be carefully sited to avoid devitalization of adjacent tissue, and soft tissue dissection should be minimized. All tissues should be handled carefully to avoid further interference to the local blood supply to soft tissue and bone.[52]

The use of intramedullary nails in the treatment of open fractures is highly controversial. Most workers counsel against this[34,60,61] because of the risk of catastrophic infection spreading throughout the diaphysis. However, recent work by Winquist et al[62] suggests that open fractures of the femur can be successfully treated by intramedullary nailing. The authors also comment that their present practice is to perform primary nailing of Type I and Type II open fractures, with delayed wound closure. Primary nailing is not, however, suitable for open tibial fractures because of the lack of a surrounding muscle envelope. Although delayed intramedullary nailing of open fractures, after initial stabilization with external fixation, is currently under evaluation at certain centres (J. F. Kellam, personal communication, 1986), this technique should be reserved for those expert and experienced in this field.

Figure 2.8 This is a Type III open fracture of the distal radius and ulna before initial debridement.

Figure 2.9 The same patient as in Figure 2.8, at the check 48 hours after injury.

Table 2.7 Internal fixation of open fractures

	Site of fracture	No of fractures	Infection rate		Amputation rate	Non-union rate
			Early	Late		
Rittmann, Schibli, Matter et al[29]	Various	214	7.0%	0%	3.3%*	0.5% (patella)
Chapman and Mahoney[51]	Various	101	10.6%	1.0%	3.0*	6.0% (none diaphyseal)
Clifford, Webb, Beauchamp et al[52]	Tibia	97	10.3%	1.0%	1.0%	1.0%
Moed, Kellam, Foster et al[53]	Forearm	79	2.5%	0%	0%	8.8%
Bell, Beauchamp, Kellam et al[54]	Humerus	14	7.1%	0%	0%	0%
		505	7.5%†	0.4%†		

*All occurred in fractures with associated major vascular injuries
†Figures represent average percentage rates

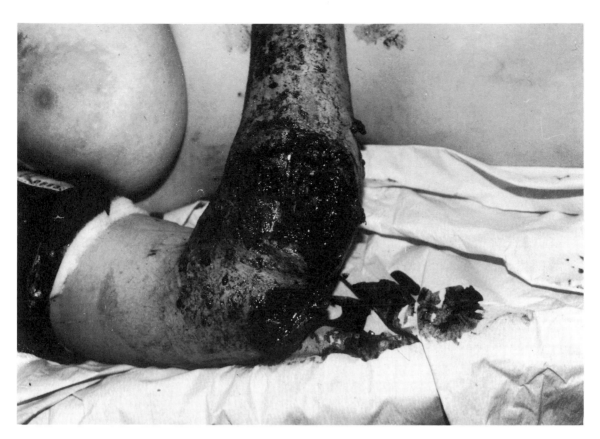
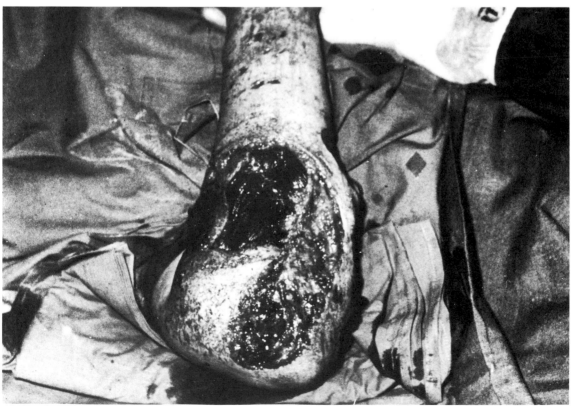

Delayed wound closure

As a general rule, no open fracture wounds should be primarily closed. Military surgeons have long advocated the use of delayed skin closure of traumatic wounds[63] although this lesson periodically has to be relearnt in civilian practice. Wounds associated with Type I open fractures are, by definition, small and not associated with skin loss. Primary closure of such wounds is acceptable, providing that this can be achieved without tension.[52] When assessing the feasibility of primary closure, the surgeon must remember that post-operative swelling may place the wound under tension. If there is any doubt, the wound should be left open. These small open wounds usually heal quickly by granulation.

More severe open injuries (Type II and Type III fractures) should never be closed primarily. The wound should be dressed and reinspected in twenty-four to forty-eight hours. In severe injuries, this 'second look' should be performed in an operating theatre with the patient anaesthetized, as further debridement may be necessary (Figures 2.8 and 2.9). Indeed, wound debridement should not be considered as a single event, but rather as a staged, sequential procedure.[52] The patient should return to the operating theatre at twenty-four to forty-eight hour intervals as often as is required, to ensure that wound debridement is complete.

Skin cover is obtained only once the wound is clearly clean and healthy, with no signs of infection. Split skin grafting is often required, but major soft tissue defects should be managed in consultation with a plastic surgeon.

Conclusion

The primary aim of the treatment of open fractures is the prevention of infection. An understanding of the dynamics of bone infection allows logical management plans to be formulated.

Open fractures are surgical emergencies which should be treated as soon as possible after injury. The five basic principles of management are:

1. Stop further bacterial contamination by covering the wound with an antiseptic-soaked dressing when the patient arrives in hospital.

2. Prevent bacterial proliferation by proceeding with surgical debridement as soon as possible and by using appropriate systemic antibiotics in high dosages.

3. Perform a thorough mechanical cleansing of the wound, followed by a meticulous surgical debridement.

4. Ensure fracture stability by using the appropriate techniques of internal or external fixation.

5. Leave the wound open and carry out sequential debridements until skin cover can be obtained as a delayed procedure.

Finally, for optimum recovery, the surgeon must ensure that functional rehabilitation is started as soon as possible after injury.

3

Skin cover in open tibial fractures

R. P. Clifford, MB, ChB, FRCS

The tibia lies in a poorly protected subcutaneous position and when fractured it is often complicated by a communicating open wound. The presence of such a wound may imply a high energy injury and have a significant deleterious effect on bony healing and final outcome. The wound may complicate the fracture in a variety of ways:

1. Bacterial contamination is inevitable, with the risk of progression to frank infection and possible osteomyelitis.
2. Skin loss exposes underlying tissues, leaving them unprotected and in danger of desiccation and further damage.
3. Extensive deep tissue loss, particularly involving muscle, may jeopardize local blood supply, upon which tissue healing and bony union are dependent.

In an attempt to document prognostic indicators and allow comparative studies, numerous authors have developed classifications based on wound severity. The grading of Gustilo and Anderson (see pages 17–18) is based on broad categories of skin and soft tissue damage and remains a useful, if not entirely accurate, guide to prognosis.[1]

Principles of management

The ultimate goals in the treatment of any fracture are bony union, with restoration of the anatomy and an early return to normal function of the limb. In the case of the open fracture, these can be achieved only by careful attention to the open wound. Prevention of infection and the importance of thorough soft tissue debridement has been covered in the preceding chapter. This chapter concentrates on the provision of a well vascularized soft tissue environment that will promote durable skin cover and fracture union.

Timing of wound closure

The timing of skin closure has long been controversial.[2,3] There is no doubt that to suture a wound under tension defies all surgical principles and invites disaster. In wounds that are traumatic in origin, local tissues are inevitably oedematous and, with postoperative swelling primary closure will almost certainly cause significant tension at the suture line. In practice, small linear Type I lacerations without skin loss may be safely sutured primarily, but attempts to close larger Type II wounds primarily frequently result in abscess formation and wound necrosis.[4] Type III wounds cannot be sutured since, by definition, they are large and invariably associated with extensive skin loss. To ensure complete wound debridement, these wounds are better left open, covered with a moist dressing. The patient should be returned to the operating theatre the following day for a 'second look' and possible further debridement.

The principles of thorough debridement, open wound care and delayed primary closure were developed during the Second World War. They remain the treatment of choice for the open fracture in both military and civilian practice. However, they were established before the development of the powerful modern reconstructive techniques of microvascular free tissue transfer and have been recently questioned by the spectacular results of the late Marco Godina of Ljubljano, Yugoslavia.[5] In an impressive series, 532 patients underwent microsurgical reconstruction following extremity trauma between 1976 and 1983, 134 patients having free flap transfer within seventy-two hours of injury, 80 per cent of which were primary procedures performed during the same operation as the initial debridement. One hundred and sixty-seven patients underwent a delayed free flap procedure between three days and ninety days and 231 patients had late flaps after three months. Flap failure occurred in one patient (0.75 per cent) of the early group, twenty patients (12 per cent) of the delayed group and twenty-two patients (9.5 per cent) of the late group. Godina reasoned that the improved free flap survival in the early group was accounted for by the absence of fibrosis making the microanastomosis less hazardous. Clearly, since he could transfer at will large blocks of tissue, he was less concerned by the size of the resulting defect following debridement than would be a surgeon with less powerful means of reconstruction at his disposal. His surgical debridement was thus extremely aggressive, akin to the surgical ablation of a tumour and accounted for his miraculously low infection rate of only 1.5 per cent in the early group. The higher infection rate of 17.5 per cent in the delayed group, he felt, was the result of infected granulation tissue covering relics of necrotic tissue hidden in wound pockets. Interestingly, although traditional teaching has no place for a tourniquet in wound debridement, Godina favoured initial wound excision and haemostasis under tourniquet control.

Cierny et al[6] reported infections in three (12 per cent) of twenty-four patients with Type III open tibial fractures covered by a variety of local or distant flaps within seven days of injury. Of twelve patients in whom cover was delayed beyond one week, eight (67 per cent) developed infections. These figures compare with those recently reported from Nottingham and Toronto,[4] in which five of nine patients (55 per cent) with a wound still open six weeks after injury went on to develop osteomyelitis.

It thus appears that the timing of skin cover is crucial. Early control of the wound by thorough debridement is essential and should be continued by a 'second look' after twenty-four to forty-eight hours. If the debridement is satisfactory, skin cover is the next priority and should whenever possible follow within one week. Aggressive wound excision followed by immediate free flap reconstruction may be the procedure of choice in selected centres of microsurgical excellence, but immediate cover is otherwise to be avoided.

Techniques of wound closure

Several techniques of skin cover are available but the method chosen should depend upon the particular characteristics of the wound, the condition of the limb, the health of the patient and the facilities and expertise available.

Delayed primary suture

A viable traumatic skin flap may be managed by delayed primary suture but this technique is best avoided in areas of skin loss. In the presence of a skin defect, approximation of the wound edges necessitates undermining of skin at the circumference and inevitably results in suture under tension, and possibly skin necrosis. Such areas, if small, may be allowed to granulate and heal by epithelialization.

Split skin grafts

Larger areas of skin loss with a healthy soft tissue bed are best managed with a split thickness skin graft. The graft is often conveniently taken during a 'second look' procedure, but application should be delayed a few days.[7] This delay is particularly important if there has been any further debridement of the wound since it reduces the risk of elevation of the graft by haematoma. The risk can be further reduced by machine meshing of the skin graft. Meshed skin is particularly well suited to the irregular traumatic wounds of the lower leg; it conforms to undulating and concave surfaces and its matt finish is a cosmetic improvement on the shiny appearance of a traditional sheet of split skin (Figure 3.1).[8]

The take of a skin graft is dependent on its thickness and the bed on which it is laid; the thinner the graft, the better the take, but the greater the scar formation and the greater the subsequent contracture. Split skin will not take on cortical bone, tendon devoid of parathenon or articular cartilage. It may, however, take on decorticated bleeding bone or bone that has been overgrown by granulation tissue. Unfortunately, in such circumstances the resulting skin cover is not durable and is constantly subject to minor

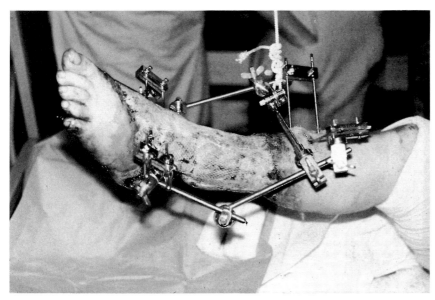

Figure 3.1 Meshed split-skin graft applied to a severe foot injury.

traumatic breakdown. Furthermore, it inevitably sloughs if raised for access during any revision fracture surgery. If used to cover bone in this way, it should generally be considered a temporary measure and should be replaced by a more durable soft tissue cover at a later date.

Skin flaps

Local skin flaps in the lower leg have long been notorious for their unreliability. The last two decades, however, have seen great experimental and clinical advances in flap design and management.[9] Previously, soft tissue reconstruction of severe wounds unsuitable for split skin grafting was restricted to time-consuming staged distal flap transfer. The mainstay of these procedures was the tubed pedicle flap and the cross-leg flap.

Tubed pedicle flaps

The tubed pedicle was developed independently in 1916–17 by Filatov in Russia, Ganzer in Germany and Gillies in England. It is raised on the trunk as a bipedicled flap of skin and subcutaneous tissue, and its exposed subcutaneous surface is covered by suturing together the skin edges to form a closed tube. After a suitable delay, one pedicle is detached and transferred to the wrist, which functions as a temporary carrier. After a further delay, the opposite pedicle is transferred to the leg and finally, after a third delay, the flap is detached from the wrist, opened and laid into the defect. Stranc et al[10] reviewed 196 tubed pedicle flaps, of which fifty were used in the lower limb to cover fractures that had failed to unite. The average interval from raising the flap to the final inlay was 5.8 months. Twelve tubes (6 per cent) were never used and twenty-seven (14 per cent) failed to achieve their planned objective.

An alternative to the tubed pedicle is the open jump flap described by Cannon et al.[11] This utilizes a return flap from the forearm to 'close' an abdominal flap. Although an improvement on the tubed pedicle, it remains a time-consuming, multi-staged procedure. Neither technique provides early cover of traumatic defects of the lower leg. Both have been superseded by the other techniques described in this chapter and they have been described only for their historic value.

The cross-leg flap

The first successful staged cross-leg transfer of skin and subcutaneous tissue was performed by Hamilton in 1854. It was not, however, until the Second World War that the procedure gained popularity. It then became for many years the technique of choice for major soft tissue reconstructions of the lower leg.

Cross-leg flaps are unfortunately associated with a high incidence of complications. Dawson,[12] in his review of ninety-nine cross-leg flaps performed at Mount Vernon Hospital, Middlesex, found some degree of flap necrosis in forty cases, infection in twenty-eight, pressure sores in sixteen and pressure-induced nerve lesions in ten cases. Many of these problems arise from difficulties in keeping both legs immobilized for the required minimum of three weeks between raising and detaching the flap. Popular methods have utilized plaster casts or a box splint. In Dawson's series, the cast method was preferred but readjustment was necessary in eighteen cases and flap necrosis occurred in ten of these. A modern alternative is the external fixator. Since many open tibial fractures are treated with a fixator, it is a relatively simple procedure to link this to the opposite donor leg via two percutaneous tibial pins (Figure 3.2). Suspension of the fixator frame from a Balkan beam eliminates pressure-related complications and superior stability reduces shearing forces and flap necrosis.

The procedure should be carefully planned with detailed attention to technique. Whenever possible, the flap should be medially based and ligation of the long saphenous vein avoided. Flap size should be generous to avoid suture line tension and an attempt should be made to cover at least 75 per cent of the defect with the initial inlay. Such a flap when raised superficial to the deep fascia behaves as a random pattern flap and thus length should not exceed base width. The donor site is covered with a split skin graft extended to cover the bridge part of the flap, which

otherwise is particularly vulnerable to infection. In less than ideal conditions, the first stage is limited to the surgical incision delineating the flap while raising the flap is 'delayed' one week. If necessary, detaching the flap can also be delayed and performed in two stages.

Cross-leg flaps are contraindicated when the other leg is injured, scarred or affected by skin disorders or peripheral vascular disease, and they are best avoided in the elderly. Often the donor site is cosmetically unacceptable to the patient. The procedure has been superseded almost entirely by axial pattern local flaps and free flaps. It is, however, relatively simple, with a short operating time, and remains useful to the surgeon with limited access to specialized microsurgical facilities, or following failure of a free flap.

Local flaps

McGregor and Morgan[13] heralded a new understanding of skin flap design with their description of the random pattern (Figure 3.3) and axial pattern flaps (Figure 3.4). The random pattern flap they described as 'a flap which lacks a significant bias in its vascular pattern' while the axial pattern flap was 'a pedicled flap with an anatomically recognized arteriovenous system running along its long axis'.

The understanding of axial pattern blood flow to certain areas of skin has revolutionized the surgical practice of soft tissue reconstruction. It is now possible to raise flaps that exceed the previously accepted length to width ratio of 1:1. More recently, several workers[14,15] have focused their attention on cutaneous blood supply and it has been shown that skin is supported by two rich vascular networks that sandwich the deep fascia.[16] The plexuses are supplied by two types of vessel—either radially orientated perforators which reach the surface via the inter-muscular septum or directly perforating muscle and longitudinally orientated axial cutaneous vessels.

Figure 3.2 Cross-leg flap with legs held in position by an external fixator.

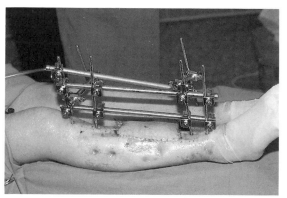

Figure 3.3 Random pattern flap.

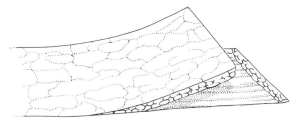

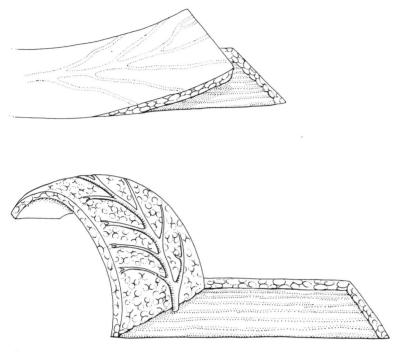

Figure 3.4 Axial pattern flap.

This vascular anatomy explains the notorious unreliability of random pattern skin flaps in the lower leg when raised superficial to the deep fascia. With the exception of the saphenous vessels,[17] the tibial region is devoid of axially orientated cutaneous vessels on which to base a standard axial pattern skin flap. Thus, to be successful, any flap raised in this area must be based on the deep fascia or supported by underlying vascularized muscle.

Muscle flaps

Although used haphazardly for many years, the value of transposed muscle in the reconstruction of soft tissue defects has been appreciated only over the last two decades.[18,19] The great virtue of the muscle flap is that it provides a robust axial pattern flap capable of introducing a rich local blood supply to underlying damaged bone. In the lower leg, the secondary loss of function which occurs when a single muscle is used is of little practical importance unless other muscles in the leg are injured. The principle of muscle flaps is founded upon the specific nature of muscle blood

supply. Most muscles in the body are supplied by easily identified vascular pedicles, some of which are capable of supporting a large segment of muscle when the adjacent pedicles are ligated. The point of entry of the dominant pedicle determines the level at which the muscle can be raised. Thus, to provide the maximum arc of rotation, an ideal flap should have a large belly with the dominant pedicle close to one end.[20]

The myocutaneous flap is a further development of the muscle flap.[21] It is an axial pattern composite flap in which muscle acts as a vascular carrier supporting the overlying skin on multiple muscular perforating vessels. Unfortunately, in the lower leg these flaps leave a large contour defect at the donor site and, following the necessary skin graft, an ugly scar. In this region, a muscle-only flap covered by a split skin graft is cosmetically preferable since it is less bulky and the donor site can be primarily sutured.[22] None the less, a myocutaneous flap is occasionally needed to cover a larger defect than is possible using a muscle flap alone. In these instances, the flap incorporates a larger skin paddle than its underlying muscle, the skin extension acting as a random flap supported on the axial patterned skin and muscle carrier.

Numerous muscle-only and myocutaneous flaps in

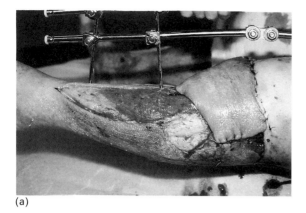

(a)

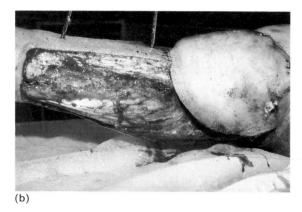

(b)

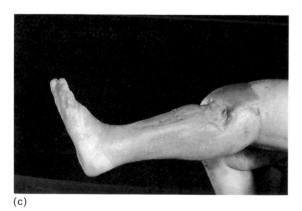

(c)

Figure 3.5 *a* Medical gastrocnemius myocutaneous flap rotated to cover massive traumatic defect of the proximal left tibia and knee (lateral view); *b* medial view of the same patient to demonstrate the size of the flap and the resulting donor defect; *c* cosmetic result at one year.

the lower leg have been described, but these tend to have relatively little muscle bulk and are of value only in covering small defects. The muscles of the calf carry considerable bulk and since they are based on a proximal blood supply, have an arc of rotation sufficient to provide cover for large defects of the proximal tibia and knee. They will not, however, reach the distal tibia, where large defects are difficult to cover by a local muscle flap.

The medial belly of the gastrocnemius muscle provides the most versatile muscle flap in the lower leg. A large and constant branch of the popliteal artery enters the muscle at the level of the knee joint and reliably supports the flap. Its arc of rotation provides cover for the proximal third of the tibia and the medial aspect of the knee joint. When raised as a myocutaneous flap, it will support additional skin and fascia, which extends the area of potential cover to within 10 cm of the ankle joint and as far proximally as 15 cm above the knee (Figure 3.5).

The lateral belly of the gastrocnemius is smaller than its medial counterpart but will adequately cover the proximal tibia and lateral aspect of the knee. During dissection, care must be taken to avoid damage to the lateral popliteal nerve. As a myocutaneous flap, it will extend as far distally as 10 cm above the lateral malleolus but the skin paddle is narrower than the medial gastrocnemius myocutaneous flap and it is not as readily suitable for covering the middle third of the tibia. Either muscle can be transposed without significant functional loss and the soleus and muscles of the deep posterior compartment are capable of maintaining adequate functions if both muscles are needed to cover massive defects of the tibia and knee.

The soleus muscle lies immediately deep to the gastrocnemius and is supplied proximally by branches of the peroneal and posterior tibial artery. It has an additional distal supply of several small branches of the posterior tibial artery that can be safely sacrificed when the muscle is transposed on its proximal pedicle. The muscle belly is broad and flat and its particular value lies in its ability to cover defects in the middle third of the tibia.

Although transposition flaps of the tibialis posterior, tibialis anterior and the flexor hallucis longus have been described,[23] the resulting loss of function is unacceptable. The extensors and long flexors of the toes may be used without significant functional loss but they are small muscles and cannot provide sufficient cover to be of any real value. The peroneus brevis muscle may be transposed provided eversion of the foot is maintained by the peroneus longus. It is a long thin muscle and may provide cover for a similarly shaped defect over the anterior aspect of the lower tibia or the fibula.

The only local muscle flap that can provide any

significant bulk to cover the distal tibia is the distally based soleus muscle. Unfortunately, this flap is based upon a number of small distal perforating vessels that cannot be relied upon to maintain muscle viability. It should be considered a salvage procedure and avoided unless no alternative is available.

The fasciocutaneous flap

The importance of the deep fascia in the vascular support of overlying skin was not appreciated until Ponten's clinical description of the lower leg fasciocutaneous flap in 1981.[24] The particular value of this flap is as a much simpler alternative to the free flap to cover significant defects of the lower third of the tibia that cannot be reached by local muscle flaps. Otherwise known as the lower leg 'superflap', it is raised by blunt dissection between muscle and fascia to include skin, subcutaneous tissue and deep fascia. When proximally based and longitudinally orientated, an axial pattern flap with generous proportions of length in excess of twice base width may be safely raised. A proximal back-cut through the fascia is necessary to allow rotation of the flap and it is particularly important to avoid damage to the proximal fascial perforators at this stage of the procedure. Ponten,[24] in his initial report, described six partial flap failures in twenty-three cases and Barclay et al[25] confirmed the value of this flap with two partial failures in sixteen cases. The fasciocutaneous flap can be rotated medially, laterally or posteriorly and may thus be raised whenever a significant area of undamaged skin lies adjacent to the defect (Figure 3.6).

Thatte et al[26] have recently reported ten cases of cross-leg fasciocutaneous flaps successfully detached on the tenth day. As mentioned previously, cross-leg flaps are best avoided but where necessary are probably best raised to include deep fascia.

Free flaps

The first successful transfer of an isolated skin flap by means of microsurgical vascular anastomosis was by Krizek et al in 1965.[27] Their work in dogs was followed in subsequent years by reports of successful microsurgical reattachment and transfer of digits in man.[28,29] It was not until 1973, however, that Daniel and Taylor[30] reported the first successful transfer of a distant island skin flap in man, by microvascular anastomosis. Their patient was a twenty-one year old male with a 12 by 7 cm skin defect over the medial aspect of the lower leg overlying a fractured distal tibia and exposed ankle joint. The defect was covered

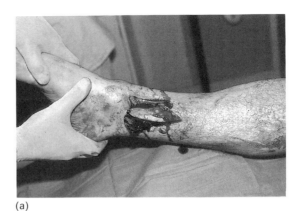

(a)

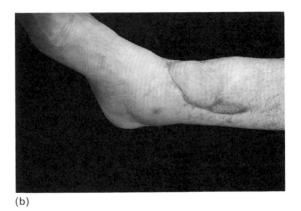

(b)

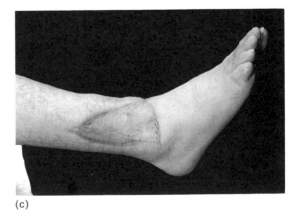

(c)

Figure 3.6 *a* Open fracture of the distal right tibia with a medial wound and exposed bone; *b* and *c* healed fasciocutaneous flap rotated from the lateral side with split-skin grafting of the donor site.

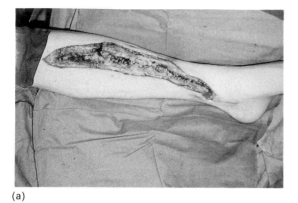

(a)

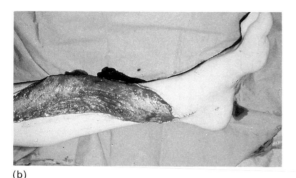

(b)

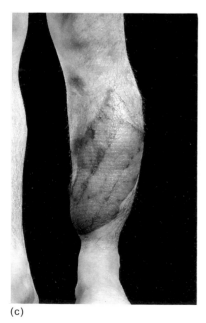

(c)

Figure 3.7 The bulky appearance of a healed free latissimus dorsi flap: *a* the defect, *b* muscle flap transferred, *c* bulky final appearance.

with a free groin flap based on the superficial inferior epigastric artery, which was anastomosed to the posterior tibial artery. The case was a major landmark in the evolution of reconstructive surgery. It was soon followed by reports of the free transfer of other single structures including bone,[31] muscle[32] and nerve[33] and later by the transfer of composite blocks of tissue consisting of bone with overlying muscle and skin.[34,35] In theory, it is now possible to transfer any block of tissue provided it is supplied by a single arteriovenous system and, as predicted by Daniel and Taylor,[30] 'the unlimited potential of free tissue transfer' has become a clinical reality. These free flaps provide the opportunity to reconstitute in one operation large and often complex multi-tissue defects. They carry the added advantages of early rehabilitation and short hospital in-patient care.

The absolute prerequisite for the success of a free flap is a healthy recipient vessel, undamaged by trauma, inflammation or disease. Pre-operative flow studies are advisable and if there is any doubt about vessel patency, an arteriogram is mandatory. Should local vessels be diseased, a vein graft from a more proximal healthy vessel may be considered, and since the introduction of the end-to-side anastomosis by Godina in 1979,[36] free transfer remains possible even in the limb surviving on one healthy vessel. Ideally, the donor flap should have a long pedicle with large calibre vessels. These should be anastomosed to recipient vessels of a similar or larger diameter. Using these techniques, most authors report a vascular patency rate of approximately 95 per cent.[37–39]

Free skin flaps (as opposed to composite flaps) provide ideal cover for exposed tendons and defects over the dorsum of the foot and front of the ankle. The two popular skin flaps currently used are the groin flap, based on the superficial epigastric artery or the superficial circumflex iliac artery,[40] and the deltopectoral flap based on the upper parasternal perforating branches of the internal mammary artery.[41] Both provide excellent flaps but the groin flap is generally preferable since it leaves a more cosmetically acceptable scar.

Soft tissue defects exposing large areas of injured, devascularized bone are better covered by a free muscle flap. Of these, the latissimus dorsi flap is the most popular; it can be raised as a massive flap and its long pedicle is based on the large bore thoracodorsal artery. Bailey and Godfrey[42] reported nine cases of latissimus dorsi free flaps with one case of flap failure due to avulsion at the anastomosis. Taylor[43] feels, however, that the latissimus dorsi flap is too bulky for the lower leg (Figure 3.7). He prefers the inferior rectus abdominis free flap based on the deep inferior epigastric pedicle.[44,45] This is extremely versatile. It has a long pedicle with large bore vessels and the muscle is long, broad, thin and flat to provide ideal surfacing of the tibia. Both of these muscle flaps may be raised with overlying skin as a free myocutaneous flap but muscle-only flaps covered with a meshed split skin graft are generally preferred; the donor site is easier to close, with an associated lower morbidity, the anastomosis may be made easier by inlaying the muscle in an inverted position and the flap is usually less bulky than a myocutaneous flap.[42]

Zook et al[46] compared the results of free flap and local pedicle flap cover of sixty-four lower extremity wounds in fifty-eight patients. Of forty-one free flaps, the majority were myocutaneous or muscle-only, although there were eight groin flaps. In this group, relevant major local complications occurred in four cases (10 per cent), all of which were major flap losses, and there were no cases of infection. Of the twenty-three local flaps, twenty were myocutaneous or muscle-only and there were two local skin and one dorsalis pedis flap. In this group there were two local complications (9 per cent), one a major flap loss and one infection. The overall survival rate for free flaps was 93 per cent and for local pedicle, muscle or myocutaneous flaps was 100 per cent.

Free flaps incorporating bone

Large soft tissue defects with loss of underlying bone can be reconstructed in a single operation by the transfer of a composite block of tissue consisting of bone, muscle and skin. The iliac oesteocutaneous flap raises the lip of the iliac crest sandwiched between thin strips of the iliacus and muscles of the abdominal wall, which distribute blood supply to the overlying skin. This flap originally designed on the superficial

circumflex iliac artery[35] has since been modified and is now more safely raised on the deep circumflex iliac artery.[47] The skin cover provided is large, averaging 23 by 11 cm but the shape of the iliac crest limits the straight segment of bone to between 6 and 8 cm. Taylor,[43] reporting on the free transfer of forty-eight vascularized bone grafts to the jaw, upper limb, pelvis and leg, documented four flap failures, and of the twenty-seven successful transfers to the lower limb, six developed stress fractures. He concluded that the iliac osteocutaneous flap is ideally suited to covering a large skin defect overlying a 5 to 8 cm defect of the tibia but osseous defects exceeding 8 cm are better managed by a vascularized fibular graft from the opposite leg, even if this requires skin cover as a separate first stage. The disadvantage of a two-staged procedure may be overcome by anastomosing the pedicles of a free latissimus dorsi flap and a free fibular graft and transferring the combined unit in a single stage.[48] A less hazardous alternative, however, is the recently described fibular osteoseptocutaneous flap.[49] This composite graft incorporates a vascularized fibula and an overlying area of skin on the lateral border of the leg, supported by direct cutaneous branches of the peroneal artery passing to the surface in the posterior intermuscular septum between the peronei and soleus. A further composite flap of occasional specific value in the lower leg is the osteo-cutaneous radial forearm flap (Figure 3.8). This consists of a lateral longitudinal segment of the radius between the insertions of pronator teres and brachio-radialis incorporated in a fasciocutaneous flap of the forearm and supported by numerous branches of the radial artery.[50] The flap is raised on a whole segment of the radial artery, which may be anastomosed in a loop so as to provide proximal vascular supply and a

Figure 3.8 A radial cutaneous forearm flap.

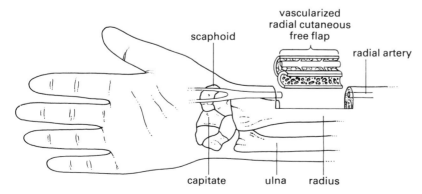

distal run-off. Its specific value is that in addition to skin cover and bone reconstruction it can be used as a vascular graft to bypass an arterial defect.

The free transfer of large blocks of tissue by microvascular surgery is potentially the most powerful operation in reconstructive surgery. However, these are specialized techniques for which facilities are available only at major centres. They should be reserved for those cases with no desirable alternative. In the enthusiasm to turn to these techniques, it must not be forgotten that if a salvaged limb is to be of value, it must be capable of useful function. Attempts to save a limb with little chance of achieving this goal are misguided. In such circumstances, a below-knee amputation and a well fitting prosthesis are capable of producing excellent functional results and remain the treatment of choice.

Conclusion

Prevention of sepsis and bony healing in the open tibial fracture are dependent on early control of the wound followed rapidly by appropriate soft tissue cover.

● Wound debridement must be meticulous. In large wounds it should be regarded as a multi-staged procedure and checked at least once in a fully equipped operating theatre.

● The vast majority of wounds can be covered with a split skin graft.

● Large wounds with exposed bone must be covered by a flap, a local flap being a simpler and thus often a better alternative to a free flap.

● To select the local flap of choice, the tibia may conveniently be divided into thirds.

The upper two-thirds are easily covered by muscle flaps, the proximal third by the gastrocnemius and the middle third by the soleus. Both of these should then be covered with a split skin graft.

The distal third cannot be reached by a reliable local muscle flap and when possible should be covered by a fasciocutaneous flap.

● A free flap is indicated at any level when the condition of adjacent tissues precludes the use of a local flap or when it is desirable to include bone in the flap.

● Soft tissue alone is best provided by a free latissimus dorsi flap or a free epigastric flap covered by split skin.

In the last twenty years there have been revolutionary advances in the field of reconstructive surgery. Soft tissue reconstruction of severe traumatic defects of the lower leg is no longer restricted to the time-consuming cross-leg or tubed pedicle flap. The techniques now available provide the opportunity to repair severe defects and salvage limbs which hitherto were doomed to amputation. None the less, these techniques should be reserved for those cases in which there is a realistic chance of achieving a satisfactory functional recovery of the limb. Clearly each case must be assessed on its individual merits. Massive tissue defects involving loss of whole muscle groups in addition to extensive segmental bone loss or disruption of the posterior tibial nerve may require an unacceptable commitment by the patient to a long-term programme of surgery and rehabilitation. These patients are better served by a primary below-knee amputation which should provide a more rapid recovery and an early return to functional activity. Only through a rational approach, preferably with the plastic and orthopaedic surgeons cooperating closely, can the best results be achieved in the treatment of these potentially crippling injuries.

4

Bone healing

W. Mintowt-Czyz, MB, BS, FRCS

In fracture management, choice depends on a clear understanding of how bone healing occurs in the absence of intervention, and how that process may be modified by any particular method of treatment.

Although specialized epithelia, such as those of the liver or the endocrine glands, have remarkable powers of regeneration, in tissues other than bone injury generally excites a fibroblast response which results in the formation of a permanent blemish. However, bone is unique in that it heals by the formation of more normal bone and, for the most part, without the scar formation that characterizes all other tissue repair. Indeed, bone healing by scar formation constitutes a failure of union.

Whatever part of the skeleton it comes from, bone normally has a fine-fibred lamellar structure. This is true of cortical and cancellous bone, whether from the diaphyseal, the metaphyseal or the epiphyseal regions. It is not surprising, therefore, that the healing of bone occurs by exactly the same mechanism regardless of where the skeletal injury is sustained. It is a matter of everyday experience that cortical fractures heal with more or less abundant external callus, while cancellous fractures, such as those of the distal radius or medial malleolus, elaborate no significant radiologically visible callus. These differing clinical observations do not mean that there are two kinds of bone healing, but it is true that different manifestations of the same process may be distinguished, one of which is evident as callus while the other is not. These various manifestations appear to be dependent on the physical environment of the fracture on the one hand, and the structural morphology of the bone on the other.

Bleeding, haematoma and tissue death

When the shaft of a long bone is broken, the medullary blood vessels are disrupted, the periosteum is often torn, and surrounding muscle and other soft tissues are usually damaged. The consequence is that the bone of the fracture ends is initially surrounded by some haematoma and a variable amount of dead or damaged soft tissue. At the same time as the medullary blood supply is disrupted, the capillaries that run the length of the Haversian systems of the cortex are also torn. Clot forms within them and deprives the local osteocytes of their route for metabolic exchange. These oesteocytes die, and with them dies a variable amount of bone in the parts of the fracture fragments that are closest to the fracture plane. These dead bone ends may have important mechanical functions, but cannot participate directly in the cellular events that lead to the formation of callus. In cortical bone, the prime determinant of the extent of bone death is the energy expended in the process of injury. High energy injury is associated with severe comminution and extensive soft tissue injury, both of which devitalize large volumes of bone. The blood supply of cancellous bone is richer than that of cortical bone, and the architecture of the trabeculae and their supporting vasculature is such that bone death is far less extensive in cancellous fractures.

The injury around a fracture excites an immediate inflammatory response which is attended by the accumulation of leucocytes and macrophages effecting a resolution of the haematoma and the removal of dead tissue. Healing of the soft parts is prefaced by the formation of vascular granulations in association with fibroblasts, with the eventual formation of scar. Although the cellular activity related to this scarring process is not directly concerned with the healing of bone as such, it occurs at the same time and in the same region, and it is necessary to the support of the process of bone healing.

Induction of callus

The term 'callus' is used in many different ways, all of which imply the formation of new bone in response to bone injury. It is particularly associated with the appearance of a mass of bone peripheral to a diaphyseal fracture, and it is in this sense alone that 'callus' is used here. According to this definition, callus is merely a descriptive term referring to a macroscopically visible mass of new bone forming around a fracture and distributed peripheral to it. This appearance is easily recognizable on X-rays, and is a feature of fractures in cortical bone.

It is a truism that callus forms because there is a fracture. The point of this statement is to highlight the fact that bone injury alone does not produce callus. An amputation stump is an instance of bone injury which does not elaborate callus. When examined histologically, a stump shows evidence of a hypertrophic cellular response, but this rapidly undergoes involution and no visible callus results (Phillips and McKibbin; unpublished data). This initial cellular activity following injury has been termed by McKibbin 'the primary bone response'.

Given that the damage to overlying soft tissue is not too extensive, induction of callus following the primary bone response is dependent on two conditions, namely the presence of fracture fragments and movement between them. When these conditions are satisfied, a bone injury will induce the primary bone response to continue with a series of events that leads to callus formation. Callus does not form if movement is abolished at the site of a fracture; neither does it form at an amputation stump where an isolated bone end cannot fulfil the condition of the presence of fragments. If fracture fragments are widely separated, the situation may be analogous to

an amputation stump and callus may not form. It might therefore be the case that a sufficient proximity of the bone ends is also a prerequisite for callus induction.

In considering the induction of callus, the term fracture can be taken to imply three things:

1. fracture fragments

2. a sufficient degree of fragment proximity

3. the presence of movement between the fragments.

If any of these is lacking, callus may not form despite an initial primary bone response to injury.

Phases of callus

There have been several attempts to classify fracture healing into various stages based on histological appearance. However, these descriptions are not particularly helpful clinically, and have little relevance to what the surgeon feels in his hands when he examines a patient with a fracture. The following scheme seeks to correlate biological events with clinical experience. It is much less a chronological series than a framework of clinical observation.

Callus may be said to evolve in three phases. The first of these is the cellular phase, which is characterized by the rapid accumulation of a large mass of mesenchyme-derived cells about the injured parts. This cellular callus is radiologically invisible, but is easily felt clinically as a mass of solid tissue ensheathing the fracture (the fracture becomes 'sticky'). It is particularly felt in the clavicle where it is superficial, and in the femur where it is commonly massive.

The second phase is mineralized, visible on X-rays, and it is dependent on the accumulation of mineral in the chondroid and osteoid ground substance elaborated by the cells of the cellular callus. It seems that the onset of mineralization may be dependent on the conditions of mechanical stability occasioned by the preliminary accumulation of the soft tissue callus. Mechanical stability characterizes the condition of clinical bone union.

In the final bony phase, the mineralized tissue which has joined the fracture is exchanged for lamellar bone which, for the most part, takes up the morphological variety of compact Haversian bone. The bone fragments have yet to be reconstituted into something resembling normal diaphyseal bone. In particular, lamellar bone must take the place of woven bone, and osteonal Haversian systems are required to restore the capacity for normal function. This final bony stage corresponds to the period of radiological consolidation.

Cellular callus

Within a few days of injury, an accumulation of mesenchymal-looking cells is evident around the fracture (Figure 4.1). Where these cells come from has long been an issue for speculation and investigation. Some undoubtedly arise from the osteogenic rest cells of the deep surface, or cambial layer, of the periosteum. These cells can be seen to divide in response to injury, and are well demonstrated in the radioisotope studies of Tonna and Cronkite.[1] In a fracture where the periosteum remains intact, it is likely that most of the callus-forming cells come from this source.

However, there is good evidence that mesenchymal cells with osteogenic potential from other sources contribute to the osteogenic activity that characterizes fracture healing. Their origin has variously been thought to be bone marrow, spleen, capillary endothelium and soft tissue surrounding the fracture. It is impossible to discount such origins entirely, but it is unlikely that they contribute significantly to callus formation. One further source of osteogenic cells has, however, been well documented. Areas of tissue destined to be the sites of bone formation manifest the ingrowth of capillary buds which are intimately associated with the appearance of spindle-shaped cells that have the ability to differentiate into osteogenic cells. It is possible that these cells are derived from the pericytes found in intimate association with capillary walls, arterioles and venules.

The primary bone response is associated with an increase in mesenchymal cell division at sites remote from the injury, both in the same bone and elsewhere in the same limb. Indeed, in lower animals and children this increased activity can be detected in the entire body. Its significance remains unclear, but it might reflect some hormonal or neuronal control mechanism for the initiation of bone healing.

Figure 4.1 The appearance of cellular callus.

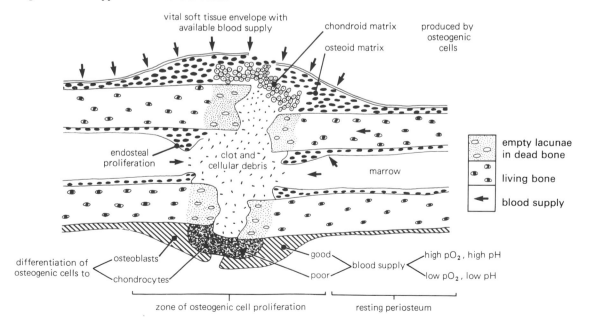

The source of the cells predominant in a particular healing fracture probably varies. Whatever their origin, these cells come to ensheath the fracture fragments and begin to differentiate, becoming recognizable as chondrocytes or osteoblasts. Their differentiation into one or other kind of cell appears to be determined by the prevailing local conditions. In particular, low oxygen tension, low pH and movement favour the evolution of chondrocytes, while a sufficient local blood supply, with its concomitant high oxygen tension and high pH, as well as the presence of stability, favour the differentiation of osteoblasts (Figure 4.1).

As the cellular callus progressively envelopes the fracture in a mantle of cells and developing ground substance, it has a profound effect on the mechanics of the fracture site, splinting it against axial deformations and, less effectively, against sheer strains or rotation. The effectiveness of a collar of tissue around a fracture in preventing angular deformation is dependent on two principal factors: the amount of splinting tissue available, and the strength of the material from which that tissue is made. Where the splinting material is relatively weak, the amount of it and its distribution around the fracture assume paramount importance. In fact, since it is the fourth power of the radius which determines the mechanical effectiveness of cellular callus, it may be understood exactly why it is necessary for a mass of callus tissue to have a peripheral distribution before it can be effective in stabilizing fracture fragments against bending moments. The cellular callus is effective to the point that the fracture is clinically recognizable as 'sticky'. This implies that, although fracture motion is still detectable, free mobility is abolished and the fracture has attained a comfortable degree of stability.

Mineralized callus

Regardless of the mix of cell types in early cellular callus, it is a matter of clinical experience that, in adults at least, no mineral is detectable radiologically until almost six weeks after fracture. Radiological detection of mineral marks the watershed between early cellular and mineralized callus.

The chondrocytes and osteoblasts that differentiate in early callus elaborate their own typical ground substances in which they synthesize type-specific collagen fibrils. Type I collagen is characteristic of bone, while Type II is seen only in cartilage. Cartilage in callus is replaced by woven bone, and this occurs by a process which is analogous to that of endochondral ossification in the fetus. The intercellular substance of the cartilaginous callus becomes mineralized when the maturing cartilage cells increase in size and begin to synthesize large amounts of alkaline phosphatase. The mechanism of mineralization is poorly understood, but is thought to involve active transport of mineral constituents and their precipitation from supersaturated solution. Mineralization of the intercellular ground substance causes the chondrocytes themselves to degenerate and die. This allows the growth of capillary buds from the surrounding tissue into the spaces left in the mineralized cartilage, which is in part absorbed directly while osteoblasts lay down new bone on the surface of its residuum. The quality of this replacement bone is coarse-fibred ('woven' bone) and is destined for further replacement by fine-fibred bone which has a lamellar structure (Figure 4.2).

It is important to stress that cartilage is not transformed into bone either in callus or in any other situation, but always exchanged for bone by a process of chondroid mineralization followed by cell death, degeneration and vascular invasion.

In addition to the woven bone formed by the replacement of cartilage, a considerable quantity of bone is formed directly without a cartilage precursor. Where the periosteum is stripped off living bone, the proliferating cambial layer is stimulated to lay down new bone directly on the surface of the exposed diaphysis. Most of the proliferating cambial-derived osteogenic cells differentiate, under favourable conditions, into osteoblasts supported by a vascular stroma. In an extensive injury, the cambial-derived osteogenic cells are supplemented by cells differentiating from the pericytes surrounding capillaries growing into the injured area. When conditions are favourable, these cells also differentiate into osteoblasts. However they arise, the osteoblasts proceed to synthesize osteoid which subsequently becomes mineralized.

Hydroxyapatite first appears in the ground substance near collagen fibrils, but later mineral is deposited within the fibres. Control of the mechanism for deposition of mineral in osteoid is no better understood than it is in cartilage, so that it remains unknown whether hydroxyapatite is primarily formed within the cell or outside it. Regardless of what controls the process, osteoid formed by osteoblasts supports a process of mineralization which converts it to radiologically visible, coarse-fibred or woven bone.

The phase of mineralized callus leads to a state in which the fracture is enveloped in a polygenous mass of mineralized tissue, which is in part mineralized cartilage, in part woven bone formed from cartilage, and in part woven bone formed directly without an intermediate state. When this composite mineralized tissue can stretch from one side of the fracture to the other, bone union may be said to have occurred. What this definition of union means in terms of the

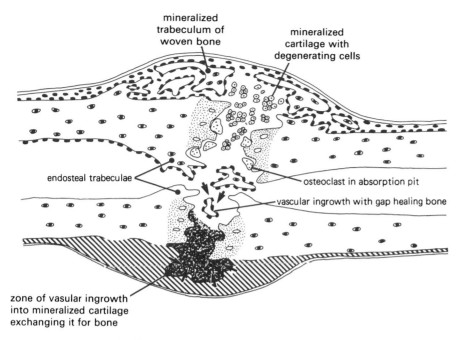

mineralized
trabeculum of
woven bone

mineralized
cartilage with
degenerating cells

endosteal trabeculae

osteoclast in absorption pit

vascular ingrowth with gap healing bone

zone of vasular ingrowth
into mineralized cartilage
exchanging it for bone

Figure 4.2 Mineralized callus.

functional ability of the fractured bone to transmit load is another consideration, for which there is no satisfactory answer.

It would be erroneous to think that, at this stage of healing, the entire fracture gap is filled with mineralized tissue. Nothing could be further from the truth. Callus has a preferential peripheral distribution outboard of the bone ends, which are themselves dead and take no active part in the production of callus although some new bone may be attached to them. The dead bone ends must first be removed by the action of osteoclasts before new bone can fill the fracture gap. On the endosteal side of the fracture, new bone in the medullary cavity seems to appear more slowly and in far smaller quantities than in peripheral callus.

Bony callus

Once a fracture is joined by mineralized tissue, that tissue has to be replaced by lamellar bone arranged in osteonal systems so that the injured bone returns to full normal function. This stage is the period following union in which the processes of consolidation and remodelling occur and function in the injured part is

fully restored. Consolidation is a poorly defined concept implying a maturation and eventual cessation of the healing process, but it must also include the filling of bone holes left vacant during earlier healing. Such holes typically occur between the dead bone ends and in apposition to the dead bone on its outside beneath the callus.

Holes in bones are not, of course, truly vacant, but they merely lack bone. Several authors have described the histological events associated with the filling of these holes by bone, and the literature has become confused because of the currency of different descriptive terms for the same thing. Schenk and Willenegger[2] carried out the definitive experiments in this field, and were the first to describe the filling of fresh macroscopic bone defects by the formation of woven bone in relation to the ingrowth of capillary buds. Microscopic defects are filled in by exactly the same process, although the vascular component may consist of only a single capillary.

In addressing the question of delayed union occurring when the fracture has already been joined by fibrous tissue, McKibbin[3] described the appearance of what he termed 'late medullary callus': a fibrovascular tissue growing as an advancing front across the fracture on its medullary side, to be followed by the appearance of osteoblasts that lay down new, coarse-fibred trabeculae which eventually establish bony continuity between the fragments.

The most recent contribution has been that of Sevitt.[4] The importance of his work lies in that it is an account of events occurring in the human. Sevitt describes the appearance of an 'osteogenic granulation tissue', by which he means a proliferation of capillary buds in a connective tissue stroma, and the manifestation of osteogenic potential which resides in plump mesenchymal cells differentiating within this tissue. The parallel between these three descriptions is very obvious: what they have in common is the evolution of new bone without a cartilage precursor, in association with the ingrowth of new capillaries into a bone defect. The term 'gap-healing bone' is accurate in terms of what all three authors have described, and it has the merit of not introducing into the terminology concepts such as 'granulation' and 'callus', which should be used in other contexts (Figure 4.3). It is particularly appropriate to adopt the term 'gap-healing bone' since it was coined by Schenk and Willenegger, and its use acknowledges their paramount contribution.

Gap-healing bone has three major characteristics:

it forms under conditions of mechanical stability; it has the ability to replace fibrous or muscle tissue; it forms within the confines of bone defect. Although 'gap-healing bone' is a very important concept, it must be borne in mind that the bone of gap healing is not different from the coarse-fibred bone formed under other circumstances.

Remodelling of bone

This is achieved by the coordinated and simultaneous removal of bone from one site and its addition at another. The responsible cells are osteoclasts and osteoblasts. Its purpose is the replacement of woven bone by lamellar bone in its various guises, and the closest possible restoration of the bone shape to that optimal for its function.

Osteoclasts are derived from monocytes and are large, multinucleate cells whose function is to remove bone. They are found on the absorption surfaces of all types of bone, seen in excavated surface pits called 'Howship's lacunae'. Both coarse-fibred woven bone

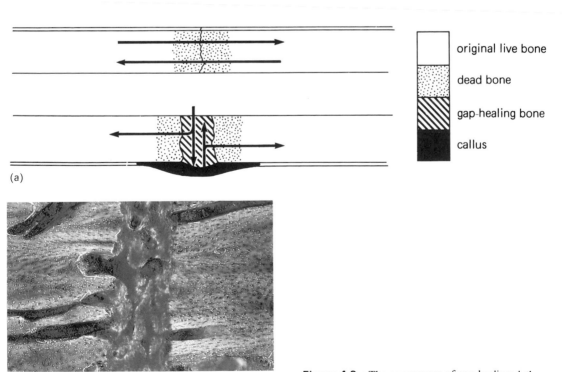

(a)

(b)

Figure 4.3 *a* The appearance of gap healing; *b* the histology of gap healing.

and fine-fibred lamellar bone are susceptible to the action of osteoclasts, which typically leave an absorption surface with a scalloped appearance.

Osteoblasts are also surface-acting, and are seen on all bone surfaces not occupied by osteoclasts. They may be in active or resting modes. Resting cells are typically found in the cambial layer of the periosteum, within mature Haversian systems, on the endosteal aspect of the diaphysis and the surfaces of bone trabeculae. Active cells deposit layers of osteoid on previously formed bone and that osteoid is mineralized to become bone. This layered method of bone deposition is responsible for the typical appearance of lamellar bone. As successive layers of osteoid are deposited, some osteoblasts are left behind at the junctional zones where they differentiate into osteocytes and preserve the integrity of newly formed bone.

Activity at the bone surface is well suited to the remodelling of bone trabeculae and the surfaces of compact bone, but requires some modification for remaking of the osteons of Haversian bone deeply within the cortex of the diaphysis.

A new Haversian system is formed when a cutter head of osteoclasts bores its way through solid bone (Figure 4.4), and is followed by the growth of a capillary loop into the tunnel formed. The capillary supplies nutrition to the cutter head and to the osteoblasts lining the walls of the osteonal tunnel. These osteoblasts probably differentiate *in situ* between the pericytes of the capillary and its source arteriole and begin their specialized function of depositing osteoid in concentric layers on the inside of the osteonal tunnel. Eventually the entire space is filled by successive layers of bone, except for the

central core which alone retains its feeding capillary. Thus, a new osteon is formed.

Surface and osteonal remodelling combine to restore structurally normal, mature bone. The former serves to remake the contour of healing bone, and the latter alters the internal structure of the bone to reconstitute the compact lamellar structure that characterizes the diaphysis. Both types of remodelling are dependent on the presence of bone substrates, which is provided by the formation of callus to join the fracture on the one hand, and the filling in of holes by gap-healing bone on the other.

Bone healing without callus

Danis's observation,[5] that under conditions of rigid fixation fractures did not exhibit callus but nevertheless healed, enabled major advances to be made in operative fracture management.

Internal fixation by plates, screws and cerlage were notorious for mechanical failure and associated infection. In the past, the aim of fixation was merely to hold a reduced position, there being no intention to interfere with the physiology of fracture healing. The use of minimal internal fixation as a position-holding bone suture failed and became discredited. However, that failure was due mainly to a lack of appreciation of bone mechanics and poorly designed implants made from inadequate materials.

What Danis implied and Perren[6] showed so well was that an adequate implant applied respecting the basics of bone mechanics was capable of holding a fracture without failure or loss of position. However, the price for his success was total abolition of fracture callus. Despite this, fractures still healed by a 'direct' or 'primary' process, that is, without callus. The term 'primary bone healing' has frequently been misunderstood to mean that the direct method is, in some way, superior to callus, and that callus formation is thereby a secondary method of bone healing.

The truth of the matter is that indirect union by the formation of external callus is the more rapid path to union, although the price paid is either malunion (Figure 4.5)—the norm in animals—or a period of external splintage with its attendant joint stiffness and muscle wasting. Direct union without callus under stable mechanical conditions is the slower path to union but enables immediate functional rehabilitation, albeit at the price of a surgical procedure (Figure 4.6). For stable internal fixation, abolition of fracture motion depends on the attainment of interfragmentary compression, which in turn requires anatomical reduction of a fracture. When this is achieved,

Figure 4.4 A cutter head boring through compact bone.

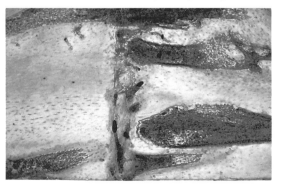

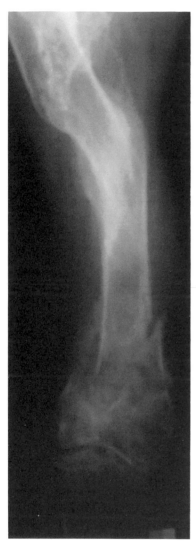

Figure 4.5 Healing by external callus leading to malunion.

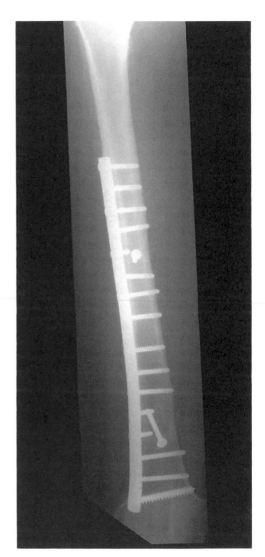

Figure 4.6 Direct healing after internal fixation.

the bone ends reach a state of close apposition with numerous points of intimate contact. Ideally, contact should occur along the entire surface of the fracture, but in practice this is possible only with experimental osteotomy (Figure 4.7). Under these ideal circumstances, normal oesteonal remodelling can occur across the entire fracture. Fresh osteons are cut from one side of the fracture, through the dead bone ends in apposition across the obliterated fracture space, and so to the living bone of the other fracture fragments. The new osteons laid across the fracture will eventually be sufficient in number to hold the fracture together, and in the fullness of time completely normal bone will be restored.

In practice, most successful fracture fixations, while mechanically adequate and sufficiently stable to abolish callus, still leave significant microgaps within the fracture which may account for up to 70 per cent of its extent. It is not possible for osteons to cross such gaps, and since 30 per cent of osteonal healing is not enough to restore normality, it is necessary for some other tissue to fill the holes. Because the fracture is artificially stable after a good internal fixation, the mechanical conditions exist for the almost immediate formation of gap-healing bone, which then permits osteonal healing with little delay.

Although most osteonal remodelling, in the absence of a fracture, takes place along the long axis of the diaphysis, this is by no means true in osteonal fracture healing. Where the bone ends are in contact, undoubtedly axial osteons cross the fracture. However, where gap-healing bone has formed, much of the osteonal activity is in the plane of the fracture, and osteons are seen to turn through a right angle from the filled fracture gap into the fracture ends.

There is good evidence, from experiments performed in the dog, that osteonal healing is much more rapid than could be expected from a normal physiological rate of remodelling, but in man it is more difficult to show that osteonal remodelling is much increased following injury. Unfortunately, osteonal healing of the tibia in man takes approximately two years to complete, and implant removal before this time risks the occurrence of refracture.

The choice—callus or not

Clearly, surgeons may choose whether or not to utilize callus in the management of a fracture. That choice does not depend on any fundamental consideration of fracture biology, for the cells that heal bone are always the same. Neither does it depend on the expected quality of the healed bone, nor on the length of time for healing to be complete, for these do not differ. What it does depend on is an honest assessment of how an individual surgeon's skills can best cope with a particular injury.

So long as the surgeon understands the biology of what he is dealing with and the mechanics of what he does, he may choose as he wishes. Some surgeons will have a pragmatic bias towards management, permitting callus after having been disappointed with alternative techniques. Others, perhaps of a mechanistic frame of mind, will have been more successful with the abolition of callus and display a different bias. Many surgeons will prefer an operative approach and combine it with techniques that yet permit callus to form. There is only one biology of fracture healing and the wise surgeon will master many methods of management to enable him to deal with the endlessly various problems that fractures present.

Healing of cancellous bone

Although healing of cortical bone has been studied extensively, remarkably little attention has been given to healing of cancellous bone, and published data are insufficient or contradictory.

To increase the confusion, description of callus in cancellous bone healing is frequent, whereas critical review of radiographs of cancellous fractures presents no evidence of callus as discussed here. Callus should be defined as a mass of bone formed peripherally to the bone margin and constituting the bulk of new bone formed in early fracture healing. As such, it is associated with the healing of cortical bone, and under those circumstances it has a definable pattern of evolution and a typical histological appearance. Callus, defined in this way, does not occur in pure cancellous fractures: the new bone seen when cancellous bone heals typically forms within the confines of fracture fragments, does not have any cartilaginous elements, and is dependent on the absence of fracture

Figure 4.7 Osteons crossing an osteotomy site.

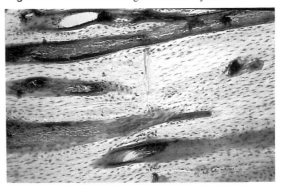

motion for its optimal development. This is not callus.

It is instructive to review Charnley's observations[7] on the healing of cancellous bone in arthrodesis of the knee. Under conditions of optimal stability, that is, under compression in the absence of a gap, direct bone formation from a vascular ingrowth was rapid and united the fragments solidly with a dense, new trabecular network. Where there was a gap, or where instability was evident, union was slower and preceded by the formation of fibrous tissue, subsequently invaded by capillary ingrowths with osteogenic potential.

Sevitt gives excellent descriptions of cancellous healing following fractures in man, but unfortunately his terminology is confusing to the surgeon. His description is as follows: the space between fracture fragments is invaded by a fibrovascular proliferation in which spindle-shaped cells are widely distributed and proliferating capillary buds are prominent. Osteogenesis is then seen to occur in relation to the newly formed capillaries in a manner similar to that of intramembranous ossification in the fetus. The new bone forms a spongy trabecular network within the fracture space, and joins the fracture fragments by interposition of a layer of proliferating new bone between the broken trabeculae of the fracture ends. Remodelling of the internal structure is therefore possible by appositional new bone formation on the one hand, and resorption of bone from trabecular surfaces by osteoclasts on the other.

In the presence of a large gap, or when there is significant movement, Sevitt describes a process of fibrous union later invaded by what he terms 'osteogenic granulation tissue' which, in turn, forms new bone. He suggests that this initial fibrous union permits sufficient stability for the subsequent formation of bone, and this is probably true.

The similarity between Charnley's original observations on the knee in arthrodesis and those of Sevitt on fracture healing is striking. Although the macroscopic and radiological manifestations of fracture healing are different in cancellous and cortical bone, the biology is the same in each, in much the same way as different mechanical conditions of diaphyseal fracture healing lead to different manifestations of the same biological process.

Non-union

Both cortical and cancellous fractures may be subject to failure of union. Cancellous non-union is not a serious biological problem, unless the joint surface is involved, and readily responds to sound internal fixation with or without a bone graft. Diaphyseal non-union is more common and its aetiology and treatment are widely misunderstood.

Charnley described the appearance of ununited cancellous bone and his observations have been confirmed by Sevitt. Both describe a firm, fibrous tissue that joins the fracture ends and confers on the fragment a considerable degree of mechanical stability. This relative stability derives from the large cross-sectional area of metaphyseal fractures generally, and from the short lever arms of the forces acting across the fracture fragments in consequence of their close proximity to joints. This is compatible with a degree of function, and is conducive to the eventual replacement of the fibrous union by osteogenic granulation under conditions of sufficient stability.

In cortical bone, two patterns of non-union are readily distinguished. First, the radiological appearance lacks evidence of external callus and the bone ends appear rounded and sclerotic. In time, the bone scan becomes cold, signifying the absence of further reparative effort at the fracture site. This is termed atrophic non-union.

The second kind of non-union is associated with the appearance of abundant callus on X-ray, with the classical shape of an elephant's foot on each side of the fracture. In spite of this vigorous callus response, a lucent line persists in the interfragmentary interval and the bone scan remains hot for years. Such changes are characteristic of hypertrophic non-union.

The essential difference between the two types is that the former represents a failure of callus response due to a defect in its induction or to its premature involution; the latter represents a continuing bone response which fails to join the fragments because of mechanical instability at the fracture site. In the first case the failure is biological, and in the second it is mechanical.

The treatment of atrophic non-union requires a new stimulus to fracture healing as well as a tissue environment suitable for the evolution of new bone. It is an important observation that atrophic non-union often follows a high energy injury in which there is a lot of soft tissue destruction and the vascularity of the fracture area is severely compromised. Once soft tissue healing is complete, reactivation of the healing process may be achieved by surgical bone injury (Phemister) and the addition of a bone graft. The latter has osteoinductive potential and also provides a physical scaffold across the fracture.

In hypertrophic non-union, the lucent gap is typically filled with cartilage. It requires only the addition of stability to permit cartilage calcification and its subsequent rapid replacement by bone. Union is predictable after rigid fixation and bone grafting is not needed (Figure 4.8).

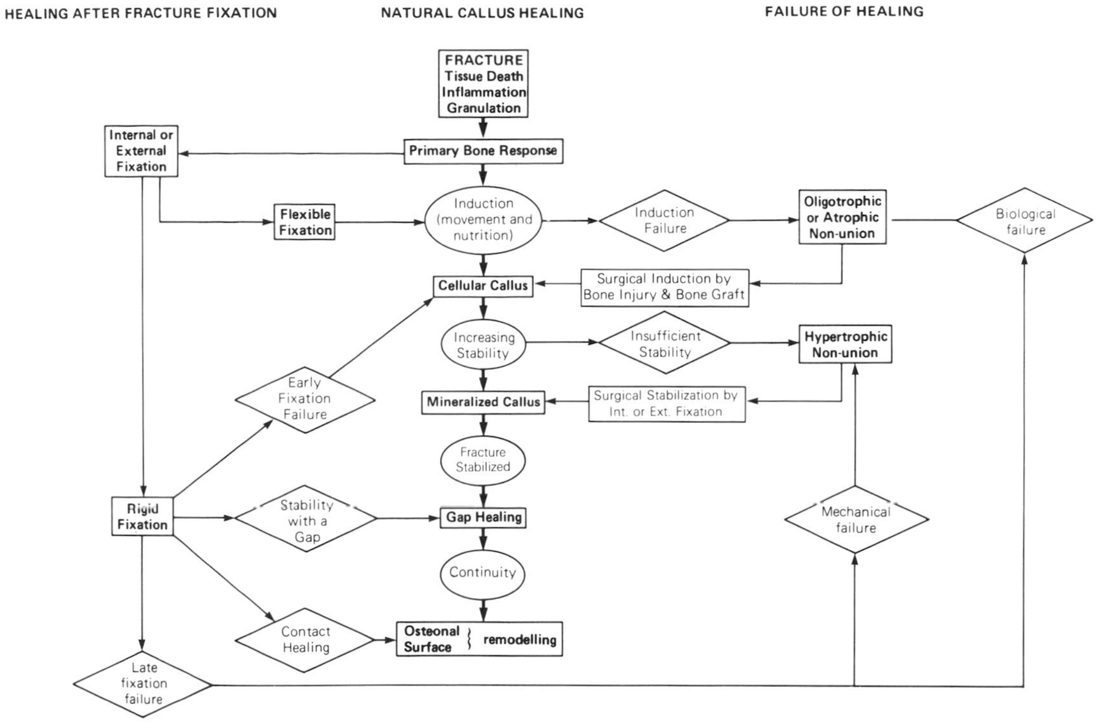

HEALING AFTER FRACTURE FIXATION   NATURAL CALLUS HEALING   FAILURE OF HEALING

Figure 4.8 Algorithm of fracture healing.

Conclusion

Bone is unique among tissue, its healing being accomplished by the evolution of new normal bone tissue. Whatever the morphology of bone, the biological processes of healing are invariable, although the manifestations of those processes vary depending on the physical circumstances of fracture.

1. Bone forms in only one of two ways: either by a process analogous to endochondral ossification in which cartilage first mineralizes and is then replaced by bone, or by a method similar to membrane ossification in which primitive bone trabeculae are formed directly in an osteogenic vascular stroma.

2. In diaphyseal fractures, callus evolves in response to movement. Without it there can be no callus.

3. The bone in callus arises by both bone-forming methods.

4. In cancellous bone, the direct method of bone formation from osteogenic granulation, without intermedullary cartilage, occurs almost exclusively.

5. Gap healing is a manifestation of the same direct kind of bone formation as heals cancellous bone. Whatever the kind of fracture, woven or coarse-fibred bone is the first to form, replaced by the fine-fibred bone typifying mature lamellar bone.

6. The processes of remodelling and consolidation are basically the same, regardless of the location of a fracture in bone.

5

Bone grafting following trauma

D. A. Clement, BSc, PhD, FRCS

The surgeon dealing with fractures must be conversant with bone grafting techniques and should be aware of the materials available and the indications for their use. The basic principles involved in bone grafting are well established. This chapter attempts to define the ideal bone graft and discusses the merits of the available materials. Guidance is given on the indications for bone grafting following fractures, together with aspects of technique that may be valuable.

Historical background

Bone grafting began in the last century (Ollier 1867,[1] MacEwen[2] 1881), but was an uncommon procedure reserved for the severe, late complications of fracture management such as non-union and osteomyelitis. Many of the pioneers used cortical bone to bridge bony defects. The strength of the bone was exploited by the use of carefully shaped 'cabinet makers'' joints with correspondingly contoured surfaces of the recipient bone. This provided mechanical stability together with bridging of the bony defect (Hey Groves 1918–19).[3] Surgeons disagreed on the biological contribution towards osteogenesis made by cortical bone. The 'vital' school of Ollier believed that bone graft survived transplantation; the 'non-vital' school of Barth[4] maintained that transplanted bone represented dead tissue which acted only as a scaffold to support the osteogenic activity of locally derived cells. As knowledge of cell function became more advanced, surgeons began to realize that different elements of bone had varying osteogenic potential when transplanted. Axhausen[5] presented the more sophisticated view that the periosteum of the transplanted bone contributed to the osteogenesis whereas the cortical bone died. He believed that there were two phases of osteogenesis following grafting: the first due to propagation of the transplanted cells and the second based on bone producing cells derived from the host tissues by morphogenesis.

In 1931, Phemister[6] used this concept when he introduced osteoperiosteal strips as a means of bridging defects in long bones. His grafting technique exploited the osteogenic potential of the bone and periosteum that were not required to add stability to the fracture. The accuracy of Axhausen's and Phemister's observations that periosteum is a more potent stimulator of osteogenesis than cortical bone has been confirmed by a recent series of animal experiments reported by Gray and Elves.[7]

In 1941, Mowlem,[8,9] a plastic surgeon, first recognized the potential of cancellous bone as a graft. He pointed to its rapid incorporation when used in facial reconstruction and recognized how resistant it was to infection. He later demonstrated that these properties of cancellous bone made it an excellent choice as a bone graft in the management of cortical defects in long bones.

Little experimental work has been carried out on cancellous bone graft in recent years, and it seems clear that most surgeons regard this material as the most potent stimulator of osteogenesis in clinical practice.[10] Recent reasearch and development has concentrated on solving the problem posed by large defects in bone. The development of the operating microscope, which has led to advances in surgical technique, has made possible the bulk transfer of tissue based on anatomically defined vascular pedicles, either with or without vascular anastomosis. The widespread interest in microsurgery has allowed the rapid establishment of ground rules for its use following bone injury.

Harvesting bone to use as an autograft adds a further surgical insult to the injured patient, and ways of avoiding it have been sought. Allograft and xenograft banked bone, inorganic bone graft substitutes and composite grafts have been evaluated. The popularity of fresh allograft bone during the 1950s waned when immune rejection phenomena proved difficult to overcome. Methods of reducing the antigenicity of the bone have met with limited success.

The recent development of inorganic implants, which act as a scaffold, has attracted interest, particularly when these materials are used as a composite graft together with autologous bone marrow (an idea investigated by Burwell).[11] The stimulation of osteogenesis with biochemical and humoral agents is a prospect for the future that could solve many problems for surgeon and patient alike.

Ideal bone graft

It is possible to establish criteria for the ideal bone graft by which the suitability of available material for each case may be assessed. The ideal bone graft should be:

1. Reliable in stimulating osteogenesis

2. Capable of providing a scaffold on which to model the shape of new bone

3. Free from immune rejection phenomena

4. Free from problems of disease transmission (including both local and systemic infection)

5. Freely available

6. Easy to use

7. Free of surgical complications

8. Cheap to use.

Autografts

Autografts (tissue transplanted to another part of the patient's skeleton) have the major advantages that they are free from rejection and disease transmission and as a group they are cheap to use. Some types, however, suffer from complications at the donor site.

Cancellous autografts

Mowlem's observation that cancellous autograft is rapidly incorporated has been confirmed by others, and this material is now in common use. Gray and Elves have demonstrated in the rat that cancellous bone has a greater osteogenic potential than either periosteum or cortical bone. The rapid incorporation of cancellous bone is due to a combination of its ability to form direct anastomotic links with capillaries of the host tissue[12] and its potential to stimulate osteogenesis.

In addition to being free from disease transmission, cancellous bone is also resistant to the effects of infection at the recipient site.[13-15] Cancellous autograft is the best approximation to the ideal graft that is currently available, and its use will be discussed below.

Cortico-cancellous autograft

The cancellous element confers many of the features associated with a pure cancellous graft, and in many instances cortico-cancellous bone can be used together with or in place of a cancellous graft.

When the mechanical strength of cortical bone is required, two blocks of cortico-cancellous graft may be positioned so that their cortical surfaces are in contact (Figure 5.1), leaving the cancellous surfaces in contact with the well vascularized surrounding tissue. This allows rapid incorporation of the cancellous element of the graft and also exploits the strength of the cortical bone.

Cortical autograft

Cortical grafts are now seldom used except where the graft needs to be strong mechanically, and osteogenesis and incorporation are not a problem (Figure 5.2). Rib grafts are occasionally used in anterior intervertebral body spinal fusions (Figure 5.3); under these circumstances, the rib acts as a cortical graft because the cancellous bone of the rib is sequestered from the local blood supply. These grafts suffer from poor osteogenic potential and slow incorporation. Where prolonged support is required, slow incorporation

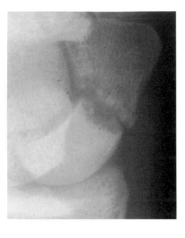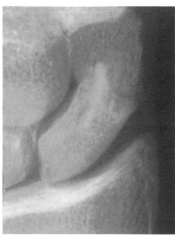

Figure 5.1 A Russe scaphoid graft using a sandwich of cortico-cancellous grafts.

may be an advantage because the loss of strength associated with revascularization is delayed.

Mass tissue transfer based on a vascular pedicle

Advances in the understanding of local blood flow have allowed the identification of areas of tissue that can survive on the arterial supply and drainage of a single artery and vein. This has stimulated interest in local anatomy, resulting in the description of several 'pedicled flaps'. In certain flaps the vascular pedicle is capable of supporting bone as well as a variable amount of soft tissue, and this has enabled vascularized bone to be transplanted from one site to another to bridge defects.

Pedicled grafts have been used in the management of trauma in two ways:

1. The graft can be mobilized on its vascular pedicle and swung into place at a neighbouring site without the vessels being divided. This procedure has been used for the fibula,[16] the proximal femur based on quadratus femoris,[17] and the iliac crest based on the deep circumflex iliac vessels.[18]

2. Free tissue transfers can be performed by the vascular pedicle being transected and the vessels reattached at a distant site with anastomosis under high magnification. Bone can thus be transferred from ribs, the fibula[19] and the iliac crest.[20]

These bone transfer procedures, unlike other bone grafting techniques, do not depend on the osteogenic potential of the graft for their success. Bone transplanted in this manner unites with the recipient bone in an identical manner to normal fracture healing. The transplanted bone remodels in accordance with Wolff's law.

Both these techniques are time-consuming and require specialized surgical skills, which need to be practised regularly if good results are to be achieved. Free tissue transfer is best suited to severe injury in which there is soft tissue as well as bone loss. It should also be considered where a large defect in bone has to be bridged. Faced with these difficulties, the trauma surgeon should seek the advice of a plastic surgeon at an early stage in the treatment and delegate the responsibility for bone grafting. It is a mistake to delay and defer reconstructive procedures.

Non-autogenous bone graft

Non-autogenous bone grafts form a large, heterogeneous group which includes most variants of banked bone,[21,22] derived from other humans (allografts) or animals (xenografts). The disadvantage common to these grafts is that they stimulate an immune response in the host. Attempts have been made to overcome this problem both by suppression of the immune response of the recipient and by reduction of the antigenicity of the graft material used. Most of the material available commercially has been treated to reduce its antigenicity.

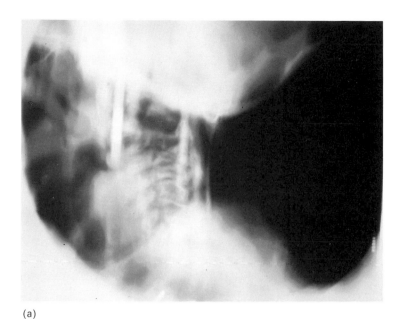

(a)

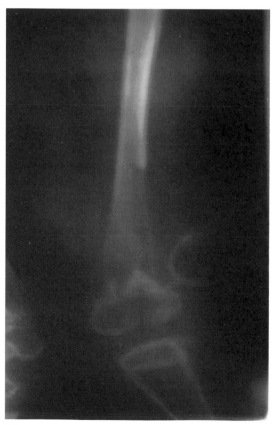

(b)

Figure 5.2 A cortical graft of the femoral metaphysis used to fuse the cervical spine in a Morquio patient with odontoid dysplasia: *a* tomogram of the graft wired into the occiput, *b* the defect in the femur.

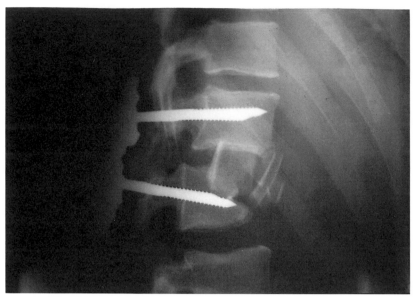

Figure 5.3 Anterior rib grafts following the correction of congenital kyphosis.

The theoretical risk of allografts acting as a medium for disease transmission has become significant following recent awareness that blood products may carry the agent responsible for the acquired immune deficiency syndrome (AIDS). It is not clear whether the risks of disease transmission from donor to recipient are increased by immune suppression. To reduce this risk when untreated allograft banked bone is being used, it is essential to observe precautions similar to those proposed by Tomford et al.[22]

Cancellous allograft

Thirty years ago orthopaedic surgeons used cancellous allografts enthusiastically, but, with generally poor results they fell into disuse. Recently there has been an increase in the use of untreated allograft bone obtained from femoral heads removed during hip replacements, femoral head replacement surgery, and recovered from cadavers and stored at low temperatures. Great care must be taken when a large number of donors are involved. Thorough screening of the donors for transmissible disease is essential, and should include a check on their HIV status. Stored cancellous allograft does not have the same osteogenic potential as fresh cancellous autograft, and

should be used only when autograft is unavailable in sufficient quantity or quality for the grafting procedure to be performed.

Bank bone

A full account of bank bone procedures is beyond the scope of this chapter (see Burwell,[23,24] Salama,[25] Friedlaender,[21] Tomford et al[22] for an overview of the subject).

Allografts

There have been attempts to reduce or eliminate two of the major disadvantages that complicate the use of fresh allograft, and a number of treated banked bone grafting materials are available:

1. **AAA bone** (antigen extracted, autodigested alloimplant) This was developed by Urist[26] from cortical allograft, by a process involving five biochemical stages in which the antigenicity is reduced and the bone is chemosterilized in a way that retains its osteoinductive potential.

2. **Pinderfields bone** This is produced by the tissue products department at Pinderfields Hospital, Wakefield, Yorkshire. The allograft bone is treated by a three stage process, including lyophilization (freeze drying) to reduce its antigenicity and eliminate the danger of disease transmission.

Xenografts

1. **Kiel bone** This is prepared from the bone of calves by freeze drying, and is commercially available.

2. **Surgibone** A similar preparation to Kiel bone is available in the United States.

None of these preparations has osteogenic potential but they may exhibit some osteoinductive properties. They have the disadvantage of an aggressive immune response directed against them by the host tissues. They act as bone substitutes.

Bone graft substitutes not derived from bone

Certain organic and inorganic materials which act as substitutes for the scaffold function of a bone graft have recently been produced. They allow bone forming cells, derived from the local tissues or added as a composite graft (see below), to stimulate osteogenesis and supply some measure of spatial control over the process. They contribute neither osteogenic nor osteoinductive activity and are unlikely to be successful as grafting materials when used in isolation. Encouraging results have been obtained from these materials used in combination with an osteogenic agent, such as bone marrow, or with an osteoinductive agent such as bone morphogenic protein (BMP). Although these materials have been used clinically, they should still be considered experimental.

Composite grafts

Burwell[27] recognized that marrow autografts contained osteogenic cells that may be combined with inert grafting materials to form a composite. The original autograft marrow and cancellous bank bone resulted in a graft with osteogenic activity. This phenomenon has been observed in composites of autogenous bone marrow and many of the inert materials described above.

Osteoinductive agents

The ability to induce osteogenesis in the host tissues has been recognized in a number of implants and agents, including allograft bone and urothelium,[28] and with humoral and biochemical agents including factor XIII[29] and BMP.[30,31]

Humoral and biochemical stimulators of osteogenesis

Urist has identified a 'bone morphogenic protein' which stimulates the osteoprogenitor cells of the host to make bone when it is added to the tissues. This agent has been extracted from bovine bone and has produced encouraging results in small-scale uncontrolled clinical trials. The agent has been isolated but has not been purified or characterized chemically. It has a molecular weight of the order of 17–18kD. The true nature of this agent must remain in doubt until it has been fully characterized and assessed.

Criteria for bone graft materials

The grafting material which approximates most nearly to the criteria of the ideal bone graft is cancellous autograft, and this is to be recommended for use wherever possible. When the supply of cancellous graft is insufficient, it may become necessary to use banked bone. Under these circumstances the surgeon would be wise to combine a marrow autograft with the banked bone as a composite graft if osteogenic activity is desirable. In the future, bioinert materials and BMP may provide alternatives to cancellous autograft as the most suitable grafting material.

The use of cancellous autograft following trauma

Having established that fresh, cancellous, autogenous bone is the best form of graft available, we must use it to maximum advantage. The osteogenic potential of cancellous bone stems from its viable cells. Burwell has stated that 'cancellous bone supplies a large number of osteogenic or potentially osteogenic cells' when used as a graft, but that only a small number of cells survive transplantation. It is important that the surgeon takes every step to prevent damage to these cells when procuring, handling and placing the graft.

Requirements of a bone graft

Before selecting the donor material for a bone grafting procedure, the surgeon must assess the local requirements of the tissues. In some circumstances, the osteogenic potential of the graft is the prime consideration (for example, in bone loss following a fracture of a long bone), in others the graft is required to contribute mechanical support (when a graft is to support an articular reconstruction). In the second case, the osteogenic potential of the graft is often irrelevant.

Selecting the donor site

Possible requirements for bone grafting must be anticipated when any form of surgical management of a fracture is planned. The presence and position of a tourniquet should be taken into account when the donor site is selected.

Burwell introduced the concept of two grades of cancellous graft in the adult: first order, containing red marrow with a high osteogenic potential, and second order, containing fatty marrow which inhibits osteogenesis (Figure 5.4).

First order graft should be employed wherever possible in operations on fractures. In the lower limb of an adult, cancellous bone is usually abundant and easily obtained (Table 5.1). Great care must be exercised to protect the vulnerable growth plate when cancellous bone is harvested from metaphyseal sites in children.

In the upper limb, it is difficult to find cancellous bone in sufficient quantities for any but the smallest grafting procedures (Table 5.2). It is important always to prepare a donor site in the pelvis or in the lower limb before embarking upon a procedure in the upper limb which may require a graft.

Very rarely, a patient with multiple injuries will require amputation of a limb as well as internal fixation of other fractures. Before disposing of the amputated limb, the surgeon should obtain as much split skin and cancellous bone as possible so that no further grafts of skin or bone need be taken.

Surgical technique in bone graft harvesting

The donor site should be selected before surgery is started, and the patient positioned on the table so as to allow adequate access to the site. Skin preparation should be meticulous to avoid contamination of the donor site, which is as serious as contamination of the fracture site.

The skin and soft tissues must be handled gently, and when the bone is encountered, the cancellous graft should be removed using an atraumatic technique. Instruments must be sharp and used with care.

Figure 5.4 Donor sites for autograft bone.

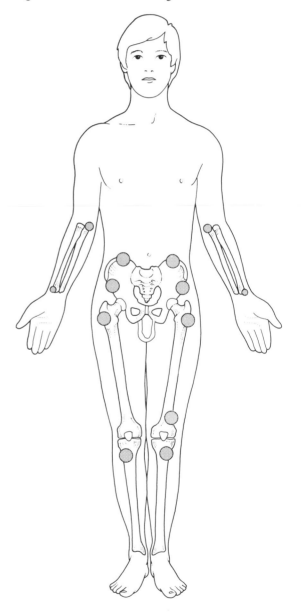

Table 5.1 Donor sites (lower limb)

a.	Pelvis	1st order
	Anterior iliac crest	
	Posterior iliac crest	
b.	Greater trochanter	1st order
c.	Femoral condyles	2nd order
d.	Tibial metaphysis	2nd order
e.	Medial malleolus	2nd order

Table 5.2 Donor sites (upper limb)

f.	Olecronon	2nd order
g.	Radial styloid	2nd order

Wound closure should be carried out carefully in layers over suction drains.

Care of the bone graft

The cells of the graft are delicate and have been cut off from their blood supply. Most cells die, but many will survive if treated with respect. It is important to avoid delay between harvesting the graft and placing it at the recipient site. Some delay is often unavoidable. During this period it is essential to prevent desiccation of the graft. This is best achieved by placing the graft in a container with a well fitting lid or by covering the graft with a moist surgical swab so that the graft lies exposed to humid air. A layer of blood or serum covering the graft may be an advantage. Any cells which survive in a cancellous bone graft do so because of diffusion of oxygen and nutrients from the graft bed. The graft should be cut carefully into pieces small enough to facilitate this. Minute fragmentation kills the graft.

It is better to use the graft promptly than to store it even for a short period. Gray and Elves[32] have shown that saline destroys the osteogenic potential of the graft and that the only safe way to store cancellous bone is in cell culture medium. Under no circumstances should fresh bone graft be immersed in saline or placed in a hot receptacle. Topical antibiotics are toxic to the graft.

Cancellous bone is rapidly incorporated at the donor site. Albrektson has shown that there is a direct link up between the small vessels of the recipient site and those of the cancellous bone. Graft should

therefore be placed on a well vascularized bed, either a muscle belly or vascular granulation tissue. The use of a punch to pack the graft home may reduce the effectiveness of the graft.

Placing the graft adjacent to the bone as well as between the bone ends is good practice in a defect of a long bone.

Complications at the donor site

Problems arising from poor technique, such as nerve and vessel damage, are excluded from this discussion since they should not occur in skilled surgery. The following problems may occur in the best of hands. In this context, cancellous autograft falls far short of the ideal graft requirements, as many complications occur.

Pain at the donor site

Pain is a universal complaint. The donor site is often far more uncomfortable than the site of the original fracture. This may be partly due to subconscious acceptance of the discomfort at the fracture site, which is not extended to the donor site. It is also clear that the donor site suffers severe damage during bone graft harvesting, which in itself may account for the discomfort.

Blood loss

The use of a suction drain at the donor site is strongly recommended, even when small quantities of graft have been harvested. The resulting raw area of cancellous bone is richly supplied with vessels which tend to ooze when damaged. It is unwise to place the tip of a suction drain within the cavity that remains after removal of the graft, as this will lead to excessive blood loss and may cause severe pain when suction is applied.[33]

Infection

The formation of a haematoma provides the ideal conditions for bacterial growth. The haematoma consists of blood at body temperature, which lies outside the surveillance of the body's immune.defence system. Any haematoma that forms after removal of drains should be cleared.

Weakened bone at the donor site

Removing cancellous bone weakens the bone of the donor site. This may lead to fracture before repair of the defect is complete.[34] This is a particular hazard when the greater trochanter is used as a donor site. Bone removed from the base of the femoral neck also causes weakening and subsequent refracture.

Hernia formation

The inner table of cortical bone must be protected when a bone graft is taken from the pelvis. A defect in the pelvis leaves a site through which an abdominal hernia may occur,[35] with potentially disastrous consequences.

Acute compartment syndrome

The use of the proximal tibia as a bone graft donor site involves the risk of a compartment syndrome.[36] The anterolateral compartment is at greatest risk, and the surgeon must ensure that all medical and nursing staff are aware of the danger. Prophylactic splitting of the deep fascia investing the anterolateral compartment is a safe procedure; however, it must not be used as a substitute for clinical vigilance and awareness, as the other three compartments of the lower leg are also at risk. Routine compartment pressure monitoring would be ideal but is impractical in most centres.

Tenosynovitis

Following harvesting of bone from the radial styloid, tenosynovitis may present as a complication.

Cancellous bone graft in the management of fractures

Acute fractures

In the primary treatment of closed fractures, bone grafting may be used for a number of purposes.

Diaphyseal fractures

Cancellous graft may be used to augment internal fixation if there is a suspicion of potential delayed union or non-union. Use is made of the osteogenic properties of the graft, which must be handled in accordance with the principles outlined above. Graft will commonly be necessary in severe comminution of a fracture or where the periosteum has been stripped from the bone. Müller et al[37] suggest guidelines for suitable cases for bone graft based on their clinical experience with internal fixation.

Articular fractures

Fractures of the metaphysis of a bone are often associated with distortion of the neighbouring articular surface due to crushing of the underlying cancellous bone. Cancellous bone graft may be packed into defects that remain after restoration of normal joint congruity to support the articular surface (Figure 5.5). The graft fulfils a supportive rather than an osteogenic role, and it is less important that fresh graft is used.

Arthrodesis

Cancellous bone may be used to achieve an arthrodesis in certain circumstances. These include spinal injuries, tarsal fractures and ankle fractures.

Fractures at risk of non-union

Fractures of certain bones are prone to non-union. These include the humeral diaphysis and the distal tibia. When these fractures are plated, the addition of a fresh cancellous autograft is a wise prophylactic measure.

Closed fractures

Primary bone grafting should be used only to augment fixation of closed fractures for the reasons discussed above. Grafting should be carried out at the time of the original internal fixation.

Open fractures

The management of open fractures is still the subject of investigation. Stable internal fixation has been shown to reduce the incidence of subsequent osteitis

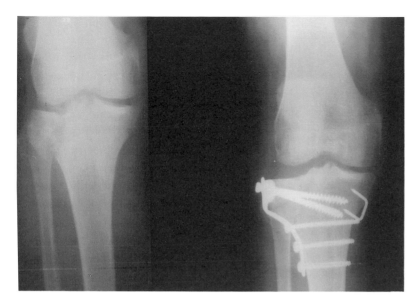

Figure 5.5 A tibial plateau fracture reduced and supported by cancellous bone graft.

where there is no bone loss (see Chapter 2). The management of open fractures with bone loss presents a serious problem. Non-union will result if the gap is not bridged. A number of alternative courses of action are available.

Immediate bone grafting and internal fixation

The aim is to achieve maximum stability of the fracture with internal fixation, and to augment the fixation with cancellous bone graft. The stability provided by internal fixation diminishes with time, but incorporation of the bone graft restores the continuity of the bone, which compensates for this. Clement and Szypryt[15] have shown that, in the rabbit, the incidence of osteitis following internal plate fixation of an osteotomy of the tibio-fibula is less if the fixation is augmented by fresh cortico-cancellous autograft. Many surgeons would disagree with this one-stage approach and would adopt an alternative method of treatment of diaphyseal fractures. But in fractures close to or involving joints, restoration of the joint surface by means of immediate bone grafting, together with internal fixation of the fracture, may provide the only opportunity of anatomical restoration.

Delayed primary bone grafting after initial stabilization of the fracture

Open diaphyseal fractures are most commonly managed with wound debridement, stabilization of the fracture with an external fixator, followed by reoperation after skin healing is complete to introduce bone graft. At this stage it is the common practice of some surgeons to replace the fixator with internal fixation. This is a logical approach and has been used successfully in large numbers of patients.

Immediate bone grafting with external fixation

Cancellous bone grafting to augment external fixation of an open fracture represents an interesting alternative. It combines elements of both approaches which have been shown individually to achieve acceptable results.

Delayed union

Delayed union of fractures is often a precursor of non-union (see Chapter 4). This can occur in either the conservatively or the operatively managed case, and requires early intervention before osteoporosis becomes a problem. The fracture should be exposed, the bone ends freshened and a cancellous autograft introduced around the bone ends in a paraskeletal site. Stabilization of the bone may be achieved with intramedullary nail, plate or external fixator, depending on the circumstances and the preference of the surgeon.

In a fracture that has been internally fixed with a plate without an initial bone graft, the persistence of a sharply outlined fracture line on the radiographs demands the prompt addition of a bone graft to augment the fixation.

Non-union

Hypertrophic non-union

Hypertrophic or 'elephant's foot' non-union rarely needs a bone graft. Stabilization of the fracture by intramedullary nail (Figure 5.6) or plate is usually all that is required. Compression across the site of the non-union is thought to be beneficial.

Atrophic non-union

In ideal circumstances, atrophic non-union should

Figure 5.6 Hypertrophic non-union treated by medullary nailing.

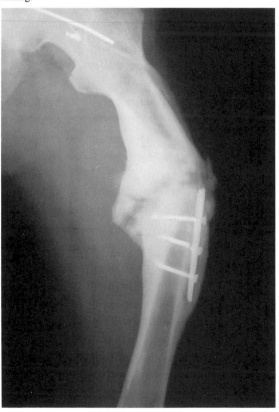
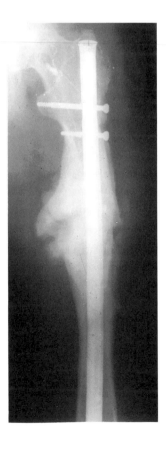

not be allowed to occur. In an established non-union, the introduction of bone graft is mandatory. The graft should be placed to bridge the defect in much the same way as Phemister suggested in his early work. The method of stabilization of the fracture can be left to the surgeon after osteogenesis has been rekindled with the aid of the graft (Figure 5.7).

Infected non-union

This dreaded complication of an open fracture is extremely difficult to deal with and represents failure of primary fracture management. The principles of treatment involve the removal of all dead tissue, followed by the elimination of infection. Afterwards, a massive cancellous autograft is applied to bridge the defect. This may be achieved either by primary closure of the wound, or by the graft being packed into the granulating surface of an uncovered gutter left after excision of the bone. The wound is allowed to close by secondary intention (Figure 5.8).

The use and timing of antibiotics during bone grafting

Although cancellous bone has been shown to be resistant to infection in both experimental and clinical situations, it is possible that this resistance may be enhanced by antibiotics. The direct application of antibiotics to the bone graft reduces its osteogenic potential.[37] Systemic administration before the graft is

Figure 5.7 Atrophic non-union treated with vascularized fibular graft.

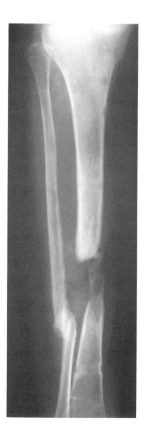
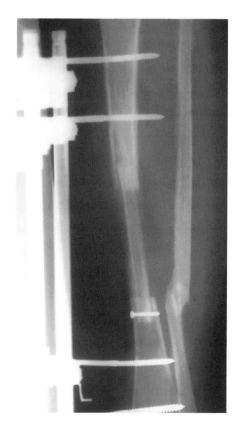

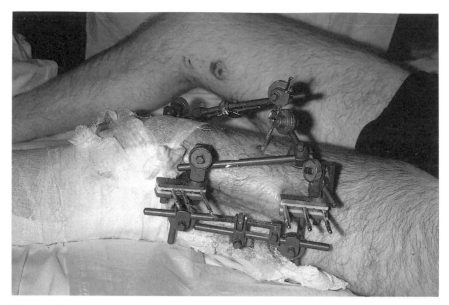

Figure 5.8 An infected non-union treated by the Papineau technique with cancellous bone graft.

harvested increases resistance to infection and helps avoid the disadvantage of inactivation of the graft donor cells.

Conclusion

To achieve the best results from a bone grafting procedure particular attention should be paid to the following:

1. It is essential to plan the operative procedure to include provision of a graft.

2. The donor site should be selected to provide an adequate supply of red marrow containing cancellous bone.

3. Bone grafts should be handled with care.

4. There must be no delay in transferring a bone graft into a well vascularized recipient bed.

Polytrauma: fracture care and outcome

R. K. Strachan, MB, BSc, FRCS Ed

In the past, the prime stimulus in the development of trauma management was injury on the field of battle. Hippocrates in the 4th century BC stated that 'war is the only proper school for surgeons', and in fact reduction tongs, traction, splintage and braces were in full use at that time. Desault in the 1700s clearly defined the concepts of wound debridement to counter the original Hippocratic methods of wound cautery. Larrey, who was a student of Desault and who became surgeon general to Napoleon, introduced the concept of flying ambulances to reduce time intervals before treatment of open wounds. He also introduced early methods of triage and stratified treatment for different levels of injury.[1] In 1878, Volkmann reported a mortality rate of 38.5 per cent for open fractures. Following the experience of the First World War, Orr promoted the use of plaster of Paris for primary stabilization.[2] Trueta later supported the findings of Orr and extended the use of plaster immobilization.[3] The dramatic reductions in mortality seen during the First World War following the introduction of the Thomas splint were thought to be partly due to the reductions in blood loss following such splintage. However, as early as 1885 the military surgeon Groeningen[4] stated that, 'If trauma is associated with shock, the latter has to be eliminated prior to surgical management'.

Vigorous volume resuscitation with plasma proteins, saline and whole blood, carried out in the Second World War, further improved prognosis and the final great leap forward was helicopter-borne rapid evacuation pioneered in Korea and refined in Vietnam. The safety of unmatched O-positive blood was also clearly demonstrated in Vietnam.[5]

Today we are experiencing an increasing number of high velocity injuries on the roads. Despite severe initial cardiovascular and respiratory embarrassment, the victims are often surviving to reach hospitals alive, owing to the increasing effectiveness of roadside resuscitation. A number of detailed studies of outcome in these severely injured patients has brought about a revolutionary early, well coordinated and aggressive team approach to polytrauma management.[6] A patient arrives at the hospital in temporary splints with an intravenous infusion running, receiving oxygen and even with intercostal drains already in situ. The responsibilities of the medical staff in attendance are now becoming increasingly well defined. Claudi and Meyers[7] have separated treatment of trauma into five stages:

1. Resuscitation and initial assessment

2. Immediate operation

3. Stabilization

4. Delayed operation

5. Recovery.

These are very similar to the five stages described by Wolff et al:[8]

1. Resuscitation

2. Emergency operation

3. Stabilization

4. Elective operation

5. Rehabilitation.

Resuscitation and initial assessment

Immediate care (Figure 6.1)

Resuscitation can be broken down into several phases. Ideally, with medical technicians becoming increasingly sophisticated in the stabilization of the injured patient, it should begin at the site of injury. Advance notice, transmitted by radio to the trauma centre, should alert the trauma team.

Maintenance of airway, neck position and adequacy of ventilation in this initial phase, followed by administration of intravenous fluids, are obvious priorities. Additional management may also include, as an example, nasal endotracheal intubation following cervical injury, insertion of intercostal drains or tracheostomy following severe head and facial trauma.

Hypovolaemia, shock and the microcirculation

Usually about 30 per cent of the circulating blood volume is lost before the systolic blood pressure remains below 80 mmHg. Messmer[9] has outlined the role of hypovolaemia in traumatic shock and noted that compensatory vasoconstriction may fail to take place in traumatized tissue. Release of humoral factors from the damaged tissue and changes in the microcirculation in various organs may further alter circulation.

Impairment of the microcirculation is a result of activation of the sympathetic nervous system producing precapillary and postcapillary venular constriction. This leads to local accumulation of acid metabolites, platelet and red cell aggregation, tissue hypoxia and shift of fluid into the interstitial spaces. The situation may be aggravated by local release of thromboplastic and other enzymes from damaged tissue. If the reticuloendothelial clearance

Figure 6.1 Immediate care.

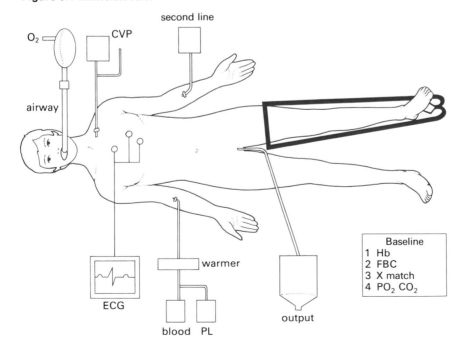

mechanisms such as antithrombin and fibrinolytic activity cannot cope with the resultant load, organ failure may occur. Circulating endotoxins that escape the hepatic clearance mechanisms stimulate release of protease, vasoactive and opioid peptides. Disseminated intravascular coagulation may then lead to multi-organ system failure.

Fluid resuscitation

Vascular access should be via two large bore peripheral intravenous lines and a central venous pressure line, followed by a rapid infusion of approximately 2 litres of warmed crystalloid or Ringer's lactate in the adult and approximately 20 ml/kg in children. Messmer[9] states that although crystalloids may give satisfactory results during resuscitation, large volumes may be required. Colloids are superior in their ability to retain water within the circulation and are therefore to be preferred for primary volume replacement, with Dextran 70 being the artificial colloid of choice. In addition, Dextran 70 improves microcirculatory flow and has important antithrombotic effects, thereby countering hypercoagulability states in polytrauma.

During blood pressure stabilization, frequent haematocrit and platelet estimations should be carried out to aid transfusion policy. The haematocrit should be maintained above 30 per cent to ensure adequate oxygen carrying capacity. If type-specific blood is not available, type-O blood or packed cells should be given. Filters and warmers should be used and generally 6 units of platelets should be given for every 10 units of blood. Haemoglobin concentrations of less than 8–10 g/100 ml indicate a need for red cell transfusion.

Following significant blood loss, the potential for coagulation should be monitored, including platelet count, fibrinogen and prothrombin times. Antithrombin III activity may be used to monitor heparin therapy in states of disseminated intravascular coagulation and fibrinogen degradation products give an indication of the extent of fibrinolytic activity.

Pneumatic antishock suits are no longer considered as substitutes for volume replacement since their application increases peripheral vascular resistance and myocardial afterload. They are therefore contraindicated following myocardial infarction, chest injury or pulmonary oedema. Their main use would appear to be in haemorrhage control in multiple fractures or for tamponading extensive soft-tissue haemorrhage.[10]

Patient monitoring

Initially, frequent monitoring of heart rate and arterial pressure are essential. Allgower[11] has developed a shock index based upon arterial pressure and heart rate in an attempt to quantify volume deficits. Volume should be expanded until central venous pressure reaches 10 to 15 cm H_2O. Messmer[9] has explained that the volumes required may be much larger than expected, particularly following delay in resuscitation or after microcirculatory failure. Persistent shock in the presence of a high central venous pressure may indicate right ventricular obstruction or left ventricular failure and may necessitate cardio-respiratory support.

Pulmonary arterial and pulmonary capillary wedge pressure monitoring using Swan–Ganz balloon catheters give a useful assessment of the effectiveness of therapy. Wedge pressures lower than 12 to 18 mmHg indicate the need for more volume. Pressures higher than 20 mmHg in association with low central venous oxygen saturation indicate left ventricular failure. High central venous pressure with high pulmonary arterial pressure and low pulmonary capillary wedge pressure associated with arterial oxygen saturation less than 70 per cent indicates persistent left ventricular hypovolaemia and right ventricular outflow obstruction.

Berk[12] has demonstrated the usefulness of estimations of cardiac output in the early phases of post-traumatic shock. Electrocardiographic monitors should have suitable alarms, and urinary collection should be minute-to-minute, recorded on the resuscitation charts. Core body temperature is reduced in shock and is associated with an increased gradient to the skin. Effective resuscitation is followed by rises in core temperature and reduction in the gradient to the skin.

Hourly urine volumes should be monitored. Urinary sodium, urea and creatinine concentrations should be measured as well as estimations of osmolality. Other routine plasma investigations should include baseline blood gases, urea, sodium, potassium, glucose, liver function tests and white cell count. LDH estimation may indicate the extent of soft tissue trauma and total protein and albumin estimations may give an indication of the extent of protein catabolism. Colloid osmotic pressure may be used to assess the need for plasma colloid replacement.

Trauma audit and severity of injury

Since attempts will always be made to help an injured patient it would seem impossible to quantify preventable deaths due to trauma. However, by reviewing trauma deaths, an assessment can be made of the proportion that might have survived had a particular facility been available. Kreis[13] looked at 1200 trauma deaths. Of those cases, 60 per cent died at the scene of the accident and 40 per cent were transported to hospital. On studying the latter, about half were central nervous system (CNS) related deaths and the rest non-CNS. Thus it was considered that 52 patients or 21 per cent of the non-CNS subgroup had suffered so-called preventable deaths, or deaths that were attributable to a lack of timely and appropriate surgical procedures. This was supported by the finding that the mortality rate for the group of specialist trauma (Level 1) hospitals was only 12 per cent compared with 26 per cent at other hospitals. These figures were highly statistically significant at $p < 0.01$. The study concluded that there was a need for immediate, experienced triage and an organized trauma system. Burchard[14] reviewed the literature and discovered that the overall mean preventable death rate in the USA for a mixed group of CNS and non-CNS injuries was 19.3 per cent compared with the 12 per cent reported by Kreis in the Level 1 hospitals.

Classification of the severity of injury is now an established concept and two major systems, based on regional anatomy, are currently in use. The Abbreviated Injury Score (AIS)[15] originally divided the body into five areas, namely general, head and neck, chest, abdominal and extremities. For each of these regions, severity codes were given for minor, moderate, severe but not life threatening, severe and life threatening, critical (survival uncertain), virtually unsurvivable and unknown types of injury (Figure 6.2).

The AIS has been expanded into a Comprehensive Scale to include over 500 separate injury descriptions, thus forcing the investigator to be more anatomically precise.[16] The criteria used in the injury scaling are separated into five categories:

1. Energy dissipation

2. Threat to life

3. Permanent impairment

4. Treatment period

5. Incidence.

Each category is scored from 1 to 5 according to severity. Scales have been completed for the specialities of orthopaedics, maxillofacial surgery, ophthalmology, otolaryngology, medicine, gynaecology and urology.

The AIS was revised in 1976 and 1980 by the Committee on Injury Scaling of the American Association of Automotive Medicine.

AIS scores from different centres could not, however, be simply added or averaged in a linear manner. Therefore it was difficult to obtain a severity score to characterize the patient. This led to the development by Baker of a numerical rating system.[17] With an original study group of over 2000 patients, it was noticed that mortality increased with the AIS grade of the most severe injury but that this relationship between the AIS grade and mortality was non-linear, increasing rather as the square of the grade, that is to say, with a quadratic type of relationship. When patients with identical AIS grades for the most severe injury were compared, injuries in second and third body regions tended to increase the risk of death with a quadratic relationship persisting. The injury severity score (ISS) was produced by adding the squares of the AIS ratings for the three most severely injured body areas. This score correlated closely with mortality (Figure 6.3).

Therefore, the ISS is now defined as, 'The sum of the squares of the highest AIS grade in each of the three most severely injured areas.'[18] Inclusion of the fourth and fifth most severely injured areas produced no significant increase in the correlation of total injury severity and mortality. As Figure 6.3 also shows, elderly patients have an increased mortality rate for a given ISS score. Figure 6.4 illustrates how this increased mortality in the elderly is most pronounced when the injuries are least severe.

Since 1974, the ISS has been validated in several studies including the epidemiology of trauma, where the concept of '50 per cent lethal dose' (LD50) has been introduced to assist in differentiating between groups of patients in terms of their probability of mortality. Indeed, Bull[19] found an age-dependent relationship between LD50 and the ISS score, namely that from 15 to 44 years of age the LD50 was 40 points, for ages 45 to 64 29 points and for the over 65 group 20 points.

However the ISS is principally a retrospective tool and for the purposes of immediate emergency triage there are several other scales based on physiological factors. These include the Trauma Index of Kirkpatrick and Youmans,[20] the Trauma Score of Champion[21] and the CRAMS scale of Gormican,[22] which, like others, is based mainly on the assessment of circulation, respiration, abdomen and thorax, motor function and speech (Table 6.1).

Clemmer[23] found the CRAMS scale to be easy to apply and effective in selecting those patients in need of specialist trauma facilities. The maximum score is 10. A score of zero meant almost certain death, a score of 1 to 6 being high risk but with potential recovery, with a mortality rate of about 50 per cent. At a score of 6 mortality was 15 per cent but at a score

SEVERITY CODE	SEVERITY CATEGORY/INJURY DESCRIPTION	
0 (Zero)	NO INJURY	

1	MINOR	

GENERAL
—Aches all over.
—Minor lacerations,contusions, and abrasions (first aid – simple closure).
—All 1° or small 2° or small 3° burns.

HEAD AND NECK
—Cerebral injury with headache; dizziness; no loss of consciousness.
—'Whiplash' complaint with no anatomical or radiological evidence.
—Abrasions and contusions of ocular apparatus (lids, conjunctiva, cornea, uveal injuries); vitreous or retinal hemorrhage.
—Fracture and/or dislocations of teeth.

CHEST
—Muscle ache or chest wall stiffness.

ABDOMINAL
—Muscle ache; seat belt abrasion; etc.

EXTREMITIES
—Minor sprains and fractures and/or dislocation of digits.

2	MODERATE	

GENERAL
—Extensive contusions; abrasions; large lacerations; avulsions (less than 3" wide).
—10–20% body surface 2° or 3° burns.

HEAD AND NECK
—Cerebral injury with or without skull fracture, less than 15 minutes unconsciousness, no post-traumatic amnesia.
—Undisplaced skull or facial bone fractures or compound fracture of nose.
—Lacerations of the eye and appendages: retinal detachment.
—Disfiguring lacerations.
—'Whiplash' – severe complaints with anatomical or radiological evidence.

CHEST
—Simple rib or sternal fractures.
—Major contusions of chest wall without hemothorax or pneumothorax or respiratory embarrassment.

ABDOMINAL
—Major contusion of abdominal wall.

EXTREMITIES AND/OR PELVIC GIRDLE
—Compound fractures of digits.
—Undisplaced long bone or pelvic fractures.
—Major sprains of major joints.

3	SEVERE (Not life-threatening)	

GENERAL
—Extensive contusions; abrasions; large lacerations involving more than two extremities, or large avulsions (greater than 3" wide).
—20–30% body surface 2° or 3° burns.

HEAD AND NECK
—Cerebral injury with or without skull fracture, with unconsciousness more than 15 minutes; without severe neurological signs; brief post-traumatic amnesia (less than 3 hours).
—Displaced closed skull fractures without unconsciousness or other signs of intracranial injury.
—Loss of eye, or avulsion of optic nerve.
—Displaced facial bone fractures or those with antral or orbital involvement.
—Cervical spine fractures without cord damage.

CHEST
—Multiple rib fractures without respiratory embarrassment.
—Hemothorax or pneumothorax.
—Rupture of diaphragm.
—Lung contusion.

ABDOMINAL
—Contusion of abdominal organs.
—Extraperitoneal bladder rupture.
—Retroperitoneal hemorrhage.
—Avulsion of ureter.
—Laceration of urethra.
—Thoracic or lumbar spine fractures without neurological involvement.

EXTREMITIES AND/OR PELVIC GIRDLE
—Displaced simple long-bone fractures, and/or multiple hand and foot fractures.
—Single open long-bone fracture.
—Pelvic fracture with displacement.
—Dislocation of major joints.
—Multiple amputations of digits.
—Lacerations of the major nerves or vessels of extremities.

SEVERITY CODE	SEVERITY CATEGORY/INJURY DESCRIPTION	
4	SEVERE (Life-threatening, survival probable)	

GENERAL
—Severe lacerations and/or avulsions with dangerous hemorrhage.
—30–50% surface 2° or 3° burns.

HEAD AND NECK
—Cerebral injury with or without skull fracture, with unconsciousness of more than 15 minutes, with definite abnormal neurological signs; post-traumatic amnesia 3–12 hours.
—Compound skull fracture.

CHEST
—Open chest wounds; flail chest; pneumomediastinum; myocardial contusion without circulatory embarrassment; pericardial injuries.

ABDOMINAL
—Minor laceration of intra-abdominal contents (to include ruptured spleen, kidney, and injuries to tail of pancreas).
—Intraperitoneal bladder rupture.
—Avulsion of the genitals.
—Thoracic and/or lumbar spine fractures with paraplegia.

EXTREMITIES
—Multiple closed long-bone fractures.
—Amputation of limbs.

5	CRITICAL (Survival uncertain)	

GENERAL
—Over 50% body surface 2° or 3° burns.

HEAD AND NECK
—Cerebral injury with or without skull fracture with unconsciousness of more than 24 hours; post-traumatic amnesia more than 12 hours; intracranial hemorrhage; signs of increased intracranial pressure (decreasing state of consciousness, brady-cardia under 60, progressive rise in blood pressure or progressive pupil inequality).
—Cervical spine injury with quadriplegia.
—Major airway obstruction.

CHEST
—Chest injuries with major respiratory embarrassment (laceration of trachea, hemomediastinum, etc.).
—Aortic laceration.
—Myocardial rupture or contusion with circulatory embarrassment.

ABDOMINAL
—Rupture, avulsion or severe laceration of intra-abdominal vessels or organs, except kidney, spleen or ureter.

EXTREMITIES
—Multiple open limb fractures.

6	FATAL (Within 24 hours)	

—Fatal lesions of single region of body, plus injuries of other body regions of Severity Code 3 or less.
—Fatal from burns regardless of degree.

7	FATAL (Within 24 hours)	

—Fatal lesions of single region of body, plus injuries of other body regions of Severity Code 4 or 5.

8	FATAL	

—2 fatal lesions in 2 regions of body.

9	FATAL	

—3 or more fatal injuries.
—Incineration by fire.

99	X	SEVERITY UNKNOWN	

—Injured, but severity not known.

98	Z	PRESENCE UNKNOWN	

—Presence of injury not known.

Figure 6.2 The Abbreviated Injury Score.

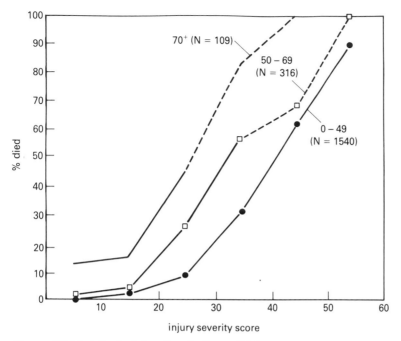

Figure 6.3 Mortality by Injury Severity Score. DOAs excluded from calculations. Dotted lines connect points based upon fewer than 10 persons.[17]

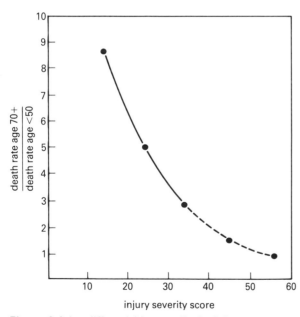

Figure 6.4 Age differential in mortality by Injury Severity Score. DOAs excluded from calculations. Dotted lines connect points for which there were fewer than 10 persons age 70 + .[17]

of 7 it fell to 3 per cent. A score of 6 or less, therefore, was said to warrant immediate triage to a trauma centre.

Some authors have now described combining the ISS with physiological scores such as these and perhaps this will be adopted in future. For example, Gerritsen[24] has taken this principle one stage further and found that the ISS in combination with the Glasgow coma scale[25,26] and thrombocyte counts gives relatively precise correlations with mortality. However, unlike other workers, he did not find the ARDS prevention scale useful. Points are given on this scale for degrees of injury, for example, for a fractured long bone, or a ruptured spleen or an episode of hypotension.

There would, therefore, appear to be an urgent need for immediate triage based upon a combination of diagnostic and physiological factors.

The initial phase of resuscitation can be followed by more detailed assessment, including serial radiographs of thorax and abdomen in fixed sequences, so that uniform projections are achieved and changes with time can be observed carefully. Indeed, Kingma[27] proved statistically that such repetitive examinations improve the rates of early diagnosis. However, there is also a strong argument for the provision of

Table 6.1 The CRAMS scale

System	Clinical finding	Points
Circulation	normal capillary filling systolic blood pressure over 100 mmHg	2
	delayed capillary filling systolic blood pressure less than 100 mmHg	1
	no capillary filling systolic blood pressure under 85 mmHg	0
Respiration	normal respiration	2
	laboured or shallow respiration respiratory rate greater than 35 per minute	1
	absent respiration	0
Abdomen and thorax	non-tenderness	2
	tender abdomen or thorax	1
	rigid abdomen or a flail segment or a penetrating injury to either	0
Motor function	normal	2
	response only to pain with no posturing	1
	posturing only or no response	0
Speech	normal orientated speech	2
	confused or inappropriate speech	1
	nil or unintelligible speech	0

adequate radiographic facilities in resuscitation areas, which would avoid dangerous delays during patient transit.

Immediate operation

Claudi and Meyers[7] defined an immediate operation as one necessitated by a state of persistent shock despite the rapid administration of intravenous fluid. Examples are repair of major vessels, repair of organ rupture, including spleen, liver and kidney, and intracranial haemorrhage. It has been estimated that 10 to 20 per cent of deaths from vehicle accidents are due to a ruptured aorta, particularly if the person was thrown from the car. The majority of tears are transverse, just proximal to the origin of the left subclavian artery. Specific arteriography is therefore required. Other 'immediate' procedures such as pericardiocentesis and peritoneal lavage may also be necessary to aid diagnosis.

Stabilization

According to Claudi and Meyers, the patient can be considered fully resuscitated when the so-called period of stabilization is reached. At this stage, fuller assessment of each system may be carried out.

Neurological evaluation

Following head injury, baseline investigations such as routine skull and cervical radiographs should already have been carried out. Neurological monitoring at this stage should include use of the Glasgow coma scale,[25,26] 15 points being awarded for the fully alert patient and a minimum of 3 points for deep coma. Features such as eye-opening response, upper limb response and verbal response are graded using a points system (Table 6.2).

The GCS profile is a very useful tool in anticipating survival over the first 48 to 72 hours. Heiden[28] describes how it may be used to determine the need for aggressive musculoskeletal intervention. For example, in a study from Rancho Los Amigos,[29] two-thirds of patients monitored in this way went on to walk and become independent in activities of daily living.

Eight per cent of all patients with skull fractures develop an extradural haematoma, which is thirty times more likely than for a patient without a fracture. In patients over the age of 30 years, the absence of a skull fracture almost excludes the possibility of an extradural haematoma, but this is not the case in children and young adults. Braakman[30] has shown

Table 6.2 The Glasgow coma scale

Best motor response	obeys	M6
	localizes	5
	withdraws	4
	abnormal flexion	3
	extensor response	2
	nil	1
Verbal response	orientated	V5
	confused conversation	4
	inappropriate words	3
	incomprehensible sounds	2
	nil	1
Eye opening	spontaneous	E4
	to speech	3
	to pain	2
	nil	1

that this does not apply, however, to the more frequent and fatal complication of acute subdural haematoma.

The majority of intracranial haematomas reach their maximum size soon after injury and subsequent deterioration is often due to cerebral oedema. Computerized tomography is useful as 30 per cent of intracranial haematomas occur at sites other than the region of the classic fronto-temporal exploratory burrhole. Besides, Hoff[31] has shown that burrholes are an inadequate way of evacuating a haematoma.

Miller[32] found that intracranial hypertension was implicated as the primary cause of death in half of all fatal head injuries. The patient with severe head injury should therefore ideally be intubated and ventilated and receiving intravenous mannitol during transit. Rises in intracranial pressure (ICP) are associated with a poor prognosis and can occur whether an intracranial mass has been evacuated or not. These rises may occur despite attempts to reduce ICP by use of steroids and artificial ventilation. Close monitoring is essential.

Bakay[33] has stated that the magnitude of the cerebral injury is the ultimate determining factor in survival and subsequent ability in most multiple trauma patients. The acute failures of oxygen transport that occur owing to cardiopulmonary failure and epileptic seizures in these patients can increase the magnitude of the brain injury. Bakay also recommends that mannitol should be given to reduce the consequences of cerebral oedema.

Cardiorespiratory evaluation

Chest evaluation should include oblique views of the ribs and repeat CXRs to evaluate the mediastinal width. Mattox[34] has reported that approximately 15 per cent of chest injuries require surgery and that 85 per cent of cases may be managed by a large-bore chest drain inserted low in the mid-axillary line. Indications for thoracotomy are an immediate loss of more than 1500 ml of blood, continuing bleeding at more than 100 ml/hr and large air leaks that prevent re-expansion of the lung. Immediate thoracotomy is also indicated in the case of a penetrating wound associated with acute changes in vital signs. Mattox states that emergency thoracotomy may be indicated in cases of blunt thoracic trauma, thereby allowing more effective control of blood loss, cardiac massage and even aortic cross-clamping.

Kirsch[35] has noted that pulmonary contusion plays a major role in 25 per cent of deaths from road traffic accidents. In cases of pulmonary contusion, acid–base monitoring is needed to detect acidosis and hypercapnia. Survival may depend on aggressive treatment, including endotracheal intubation, positive pressure ventilation, cautious fluid replacement, maintenance of haematocrit and possibly steroid therapy. However, in the severe pulmonary contusion categories, death can occur within 72 to 96 hours. Messmer[9] has stated that a paO$_2$ below 60 mmHg on air calls for prophylactic ventilation with positive end expiratory pressure.

Kinney[36] found mean increases in minute ventilation of up to 85 per cent in injured patients and he used the ventilatory equivalent, or litres of air moved per litre of carbon dioxide exhaled, to find that following trauma, dead space could be increased by as much as 80 per cent in association with an average increase in metabolic rate of only 17 per cent. Oestern[37] concluded that it was the increase in total pulmonary resistance, leading to an increase in pulmonary artery pressure, which then caused increased right ventricular afterload and an increase in right atrial filling pressure (Figure 6.5).

Total peripheral resistance elevation can be caused by hypoxia, acidosis, microembolization, vasoactive mediators such as serotonin and, perhaps most importantly of all, by interstitial oedema. Comparing groups of survivors and non-survivors, Oestern found that there were significant differences between the groups in terms of cardiac index in 1 min/m^2, left ventricular work and stroke index in ml/m^2. However, heart rates, blood pressure and right ventricular work did not show differences during the first week after accident. Neither were there significant differences in arterial pCO$_2$, paO$_2$ or tidal volume. Oestern ascribed these negative findings to the efficacy of positive end expiratory pressure ventilation (PEEP) used throughout the study. He described how the concept of significant increases in extravascular lung water have certainly been demonstrated in sepsis but results are not quite so clear in trauma cases. He concluded that therapy should include aggressive and early ventilation using PEEP, adequate volume replacement, correction of acidosis and administration of positive inotropic and vasodilating agents. This therapy, it was hoped, would help to counter the consequences of microaggregation, pulmonary emboli and coagulopathies, all of which need careful consideration during resuscitation.

Adult respiratory distress syndrome

The classical signs of fat embolism may be observed in 2 to 6 per cent of patients, as described by Newman.[38] The subclinical diagnosis of fat embolism based on paO$_2$ estimations has also been well described by McCarthy.[39] A recent and detailed paper

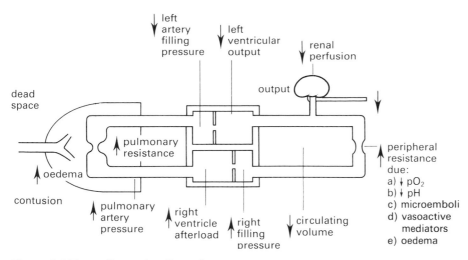

Figure 6.5 The cardiovascular effects of trauma.

by Avikainen looks at the metabolic aspects of the Adult Respiratory Distress Syndrome (ARDS).[40] A group of ARDS patients was compared with a similar group of non-ARDS trauma cases. The ARDS patients were found to have higher blood glucose levels, higher cholesterol, lower alpha–beta lipo-protein ratios, reduced circulating platelet levels, increased platelet adhesiveness, increased platelet aggregation and thrombosis. Platelet aggregation and microembolism has been described by several other authors, including Bergentz.[41] Disturbance of carbohydrate and lipid metabolism may encourage the development of the microemboli and the subsequent alveolar membrane destabilization. A recurring theme in the literature is therefore that thrombotic vascular diseases, including Disseminated Intravascular Coagulation, may have aetiological factors in common with ARDS. Avikainen also found increased adrenergic reactivity in ARDS patients and this may result in increased mobilization of platelets from the spleen and lung pools.[40] The higher platelet counts in fat embolism patients may, however, be partly due to haemoconcentration since plasma protein concentrations were not seen to decrease, as they did in the control patients.

Sturm[42] has shown that increases in pulmonary vascular resistance can occur within 20 minutes of trauma and that such immediate changes may be due to overwhelming release of vasoactive agents following trauma. Increased capillary permeability may also be due to such vasoactive agents, the situation being compounded by the capillary fragility seen in ARDS.

This fragility appears to be caused by microemboli of platelet aggregates and possibly, too, by the relative decrease in circulating numbers of free platelets. If this process is set in motion fairly soon after injury, it is not surprising to find that authors such as Law[43] have found it difficult to prove that decreased transit times to hospital, including use of helicopter transit, significantly reduce the duration in the intensive care unit. Law found too that only 13 patients out of 198 had benefited from early operative intervention for haemorrhagic conditions. He noted a near zero survival rate in those patients in a state of cardiac arrest, and concluded that immediate resuscitative thoracotomy was unjustified.

Other metabolic differences seen in the ARDS group by Avikainen[40] included decreased growth hormone and decreased cortisol secretion.

Metabolic effects of trauma

For adequate reversal of the effects of post-traumatic hypovolaemic shock, Messmer[9] has emphasized the need for sequential analysis of circulatory and biochemical factors, together with an evaluation of clinical symptoms. These are prerequisites for further surgical management.

Hasset[44] and Schmitz[45] have described the anabolic state following trauma and the negative nitrogen balance leading, particularly in septic states, to a need for massive protein supplements. Gann[46] has outlined the neuroendocrine response that mobilizes and utilizes the synthetic and energetic substrates required by the body. Chemoreceptors, baroreceptors and various plasma factors combine to stimulate autonomic and pituitary responses, including the secretion of ACTH, ADH, growth hormone, prolactin, adrenaline and endorphins. The responses of the pancreatic islets and the renin–angiotensin system may also be modified. The importance is emphasized of restoration of blood volume, relief of pain and support of organ function in the restoration of normal neuroendocrine function.

MacNicol[47] has demonstrated a significant relationship between hypoxaemia and protein catabolism following long bone fractures, with urinary urea being a convenient index of protein catabolism. Oppenheim[48] found significant relationships between ISS, initial blood metabolite concentrations and subsequent biochemical changes. At about four hours after injury, severity of injury could be related to blood lactate, pyruvate and alanine and could be inversely related to ketone concentration. However, only total urinary nitrogen could be related to severity of injury in the next seven days. Other authors such as Weil[49] have found that initial blood lactate may also be an indicator of survival. Booji[50] has highlighted the metabolic dangers of massive blood transfusion, namely hypothermia, hyperkalaemia, increased affinity for oxygen in citrated blood stored for more than five days, acidosis, hypocalcaemia and alkalosis from the metabolism of citrate.

Schmitz[45] has reviewed the need for nutritional support in multiply injured patients and has outlined a programme of suitable parenteral nutrition including doses of amino acids, carbohydrates, fat, fluid, trace elements and vitamins. Modifications to standard regimes for patients with impaired liver and renal function may be necessary.

Abdominal evaluation

At this stage, abdominal evaluation may still include exploratory abdominal paracentesis and peritoneal lavage with 1 litre of dialysis solution for RBC, WBC, bile and amylase levels in the peritoneal cavity to be estimated. Counts greater than 500 WBC/ml[3], or 100,000 RBC/ml[3] are strong indicators for operative intervention.[6] The presence of amylase, bile or gut contents suggests laparotomy. Ultrasound and CT have also been shown to have a role at this stage of management. Fairclough[51] has stated that abdominal girth measurements are an unreliable measure of intra-abdominal bleeding.

A lacerated spleen is the most common organ injury, followed by injury to the liver, gut and kidney. Goris,[52] in reviewing deaths occurring more than seven days after blunt injury, found sepsis to be associated with organ failure in 88 per cent of cases. These were principally cases of pulmonary sepsis. However, other organs were often involved in multiple systems failure, including liver and kidney. Polk[53] has comprehensively reviewed the objectives of surgery in the categories of diaphragmatic, liver, pancreaticoduodenal, gastrointestinal and splenic injury.

Urological evaluation

In a pelvic ring injury, examination should include a urethrogram before a catheter is used. An associated bladder rupture may occur in 5 per cent of fractures of the pelvic ring. Microscopic or gross haematuria should also be investigated by an IVP, the single bolus/10 minute after injection/single plate estimation usually being sufficient for reasonable assessment of gross excretory function.[6]

Urine output should be maintained with positive inotropes and dopamine at over 100 ml/hr, since the high-output type renal failure that may develop in this situation is easily manageable. This is in marked contrast to the catastrophe of oliguria often caused by hypovolaemia and hypoxia. Routine intravenous pyelograms following significant abdominal trauma may indicate the need for specific arteriography.

Vascular evaluation

Heberer[54] has shown how the incidence of peripheral vascular injuries is twice as high in polytrauma at 7.3 per cent as in isolated extremity fractures at 3.6 per cent. Temporary control of bleeding should be by digital compression or sterile compression bandages at the site of bleeding. Ischaemia tolerance time is of the order of four to six hours for extremities but less for the viscera.

Precise diagnosis based upon angiography should precede surgery, this being particularly important in aortic injuries. Selective angiography is useful in supraortic injury, and transfemoral angiography can be followed by selective embolization in the abdomen and pelvis. Sibbet[55] has stated how digital subtraction angiography can appear to decrease examination time and improve patient comfort in comparison with conventional angiography. However, high contrast loads, difficult timing and poor quality angiograms may outweigh the advantages of the lower invasiveness. Prophylactic fasciotomy (Figure 6.6) after prolonged ischaemia is essential and Tscherne[56] recommends compartment decompression before vessel

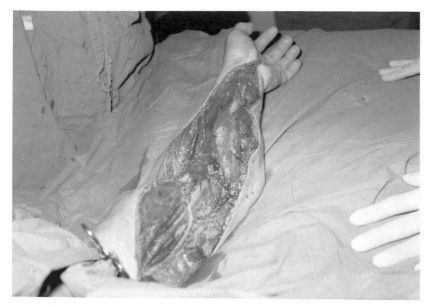

Figure 6.6 Fasciotomy of crushing injury to arm.

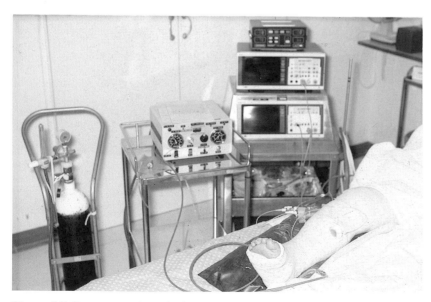

Figure 6.7 Compartmental monitoring.

repair and fixation. Intra-compartmental monitoring (Figure 6.7) as described by Whitesides[57] should be carried out in equivocal cases of raised pressure. Normal pressure should be from 0 to 8 mm Hg. Fasciotomy is needed if pain, positive muscle stretch testing and pressures above 30 mmHg are encountered. The slit catheters advocated by Rorabeck[58] appear to be the most reliable in the monitoring of intra-compartmental pressure. Jupiter[6] has reviewed the literature on decompression in different parts of the body. In the lower leg, the double incision fasciotomy described by Mubarak[59] appears to give good results providing adequate decompression of the deep posterior compartment is achieved.

Schulze-Bergmann[60] has shown the benefits of early surgery in the popliteal artery, contrasting amputation rates of 40 per cent in the Second World War following delays of 15 hours with 25 per cent in the Korean War after a 10-hour delay and a 5 per cent amputation rate in the Vietnam War following a 2-hour delay. Direct suture or saphenous vein graft is preferred for peripheral injuries. However, in polytrauma the use of prosthetic materials should always be considered to save time. Heberer also recommends reconstruction in major venous injury. Since success in limb salvage is related to the duration of ischaemia, temporary arterial shunts have been recommended by Nunley[61] and Tscherne[56] before rapid skeletal fixation.

Multiple systems

Hasset[62] summarizes the problem of multiple organ systems failure well in suggesting that organ failures may be related to protein malnutrition, which occurs as a result of the increased obligatory oxidative amino acid catabolism and the prolonged metabolic demands of trauma. Nutrition should therefore include a minimum of 3000 calories of glucose per day as well as 2 to 3 g per kg conventional amino-acid mixtures. Not only will this improve the metabolic efficiency of the patient, it will also prevent secondary but critical organ failure, such as gut mucosa leading to entry of gut contained endotoxins, bacteraemia and death.

There is today a great deal of research conducted into the stabilization phase of trauma. For example, in haematology there are studies on complement 3 activation, neutrophil function, immunology of chemotaxis and the role of anaphylotoxins. Biochemical studies have included total body oxygen utilization and the roles of the different adrenal corticosteroids, hepatic glycolytic intermediates, amino acids and ketones in trauma. Pharmacological studies have included the prophylactic uses of cimetidine and of neurodepressants in ARDS, the role of vasoactive mediators in ARDS, calcium supplementation in shock and of circulating B-endorphins.

Delayed operations

Claudi and Meyers describe the role of the orthopaedic surgeon as being most vital in the so-called delayed operation phase following a short period of stabilization. The term 'delayed' is appropriate for resuscitation, but in orthopaedic care it is an unfortunate misnomer. Wound excision, debridement and wound closure in compound fractures are essential in immediate orthopaedic trauma management. Gustilo's classification[63] of compound injuries into Types I, II, IIIa, b and c emphasizes the need for total excision of poorly vascularized tissues and, in Type IIIc, the need for adequate vascular repair.

However, because the majority of open fractures are unstable, motion at the fracture site will not only lead to loss of reduction, but will also increase pain and stress, accelerate haemorrhage and aggravate local soft tissue damage. Optimal care would therefore appear to be by thorough wound debridement and stable fixation. Nevertheless, Tscherne[64] has pointed out that infections are caused not only by inadequate excision of the wound but also by implants being placed beneath marginally viable tissues, by wound closure under tension, failure to recognize compartment syndromes, inadequate haemostasis and drainage, and iatrogenic devascularization of already compromised tissue. However, the third generation of cephalosporins appear to have greatly decreased the incidence of infection following implant surgery, even though Gustilo has shown that 70 per cent of all wounds will now yield a potentially pathogenic organism.[63] The pattern of infection also appears to be changing following the use of antibiotics, so that Gram-negatives are now responsible for over 70 per cent of infections compared with 24 per cent in the recent past.[65] This again points to the continuing need for the prophylactic use of the third generation of cephalosporins, perhaps in combination with an aminoglycocide. The revolution in antibiotic prophylaxis has occurred at the right time to allow early operative stabilization of long bone fractures.

Several studies of the polytraumatized patient have demonstrated that early operative stabilization can diminish the risks of pulmonary sepsis, ARDS and fat embolism.[6] The emphasis is on the word 'risks' rather than on the 'incidence' of these syndromes. A stabilized long bone fracture will decrease pain and associated narcotic requirements, both of which will depress respiratory function. These effects can be even greater when associated with pulmonary injury or hypovolaemic shock. The impact of early stabilization of long bone fractures on improving pulmonary function has been assessed by several authors studying comparable groups of patients graded according to injury severity score. Seibel[66] contrasted 20 polytrauma patients treated with early long bone stabilization with 20 patients managed with skeletal traction over a period of ten days. In the stabilized group only four fracture related complications occurred and they required an average of only 3.4 days of ventilatory support and spent an average of only 23 days in hospital. This was in marked contrast to the traction group, where 12 complications were noted, 9 days of ventilatory support were needed and 45 days were spent in hospital. Similarly, Johnson[67] describes a study of polytrauma cases with ISS scores greater than 40 where a 17 per cent incidence of ARDS was seen in an early stabilization group compared with an incidence of 75 per cent in those with delayed surgery.

Goris,[68] studying polytrauma patients with ISS scores greater than 50, found a 26 per cent incidence of ARDS and a late sepsis mortality rate of 6 per cent in a group of patients treated with early fracture stabilization and prophylactic PEEP ventilation. In contrast, a similar group of patients treated with delayed fracture stabilization and prophylactic ventilatory support was found to have an ARDS incidence of 82 per cent, with a late sepsis mortality of 55 per cent. Similarly, Meek[69] retrospectively reviewed 71 patients with multiple injuries matched for age and severity. Twenty-eight per cent of patients with conservatively treated fractures died compared with 4.5 per cent whose fractures were fixed. Riska[70] looked at over a thousand cases of multiple trauma over a seven-year period and found that although the ventilatory support policy had not changed, the advent of aggressive internal fixation reduced the incidence of ARDS from 21 per cent to 5 per cent. Fixation of long bone fractures, therefore, appears to reduce overall septic and pulmonary complications significantly and allows earlier cessation of mechanical ventilation.

There is no doubt, however, that PEEP has a role to play in reversing alveolar collapse, reducing interstitial oedema and improving oxygen tensions. Several authors including Ruedi[71] and Sturm[42] have emphasized the role of artificial ventilation in reducing the severity of ARDS and its fatal septic consequences, but careful monitoring of ventilatory function is still necessary in an intensive care unit since PEEP by itself can result in a dangerous decrease in venous return and cardiac output, particularly in hypovolaemic states and conditions of myocardial insufficiency. In these cases, pulmonary capillary wedge pressure estimations performed with a Swan–Ganz catheter are extremely useful as they correlate with left atrial and left ventricular end-diastolic pressure. Hasset[62] sums up the situation well:

> The patient who does not have all his operations carried out on the day of admission should be placed into an intensive care unit with a deliberate plan to complete this operative work within three to five days. The time is picked to avoid the pneumonia, protein malnutrition and pulmonary emboli that are so common with a delay of 10 to 14 days.

Jupiter[6] provides an interesting insight into current unsubstantiated prejudices about internal fixation, which date back to the days of open reduction and internal fixation. He says that, 'Intramedullary fixation in open fractures is associated with further devascularisation of an already vascularly impaired long bone'. The study of vascular responses in fractures is of primary interest; and there is no doubt that endosteal reaming leads to disruption of endosteal sources of flow, loss of cortical bone and thermonecrosis of a proportion of tissue. However, in terms of rates of non-union this is irrelevant, as the stability thus conferred decreases the delayed union rates from approximately 30 per cent seen for example in a typical mixed group of conservatively treated tibial fractures to less than 10 per cent. The reasons for this are complex and thought first to be due to the more rapid re-establishment of intramedullary flow, which has been seen to occur as early as six weeks after fixation. In the closed situation any remaining periosteum should be left undisturbed by such fixation. In addition, the injection of osteogenic reaming products into surrounding tissue appears to be one of the principal factors leading to the massive amounts of peripheral callus seen at the fracture site following closed reaming. These factors are added to the stability conferred on the fracture, allowing early mobilization and weight-bearing, which would also appear to promote union.

External fixation still has a role to play, particularly in the severe soft tissue injury, with the potential additional advantage that the biomechanical environment can be manipulated in a more quantifiable way than if a locking nail was assigned its dynamic role.

Perhaps, therefore, the only justifiable reason for not carrying out a policy of aggressive early internal fixation in polytrauma is a lack of adequate facilities.

Recovery

The patient should enter the recovery phase capable of fully mobilizing his or her joints at an earlier stage than if conservative measures had been used. In assessing the results of surgery, any long-term

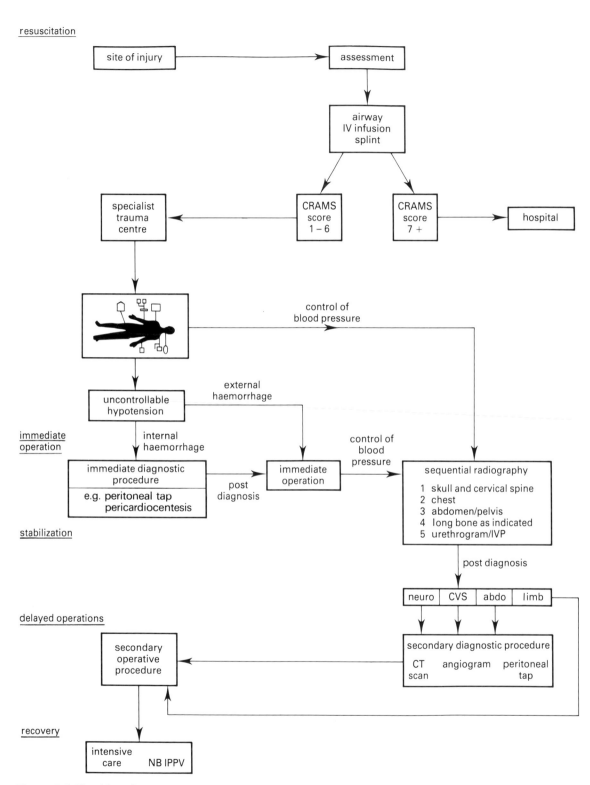

Figure 6.8 Algorithm of care.

functional, employment, recreational and symptomatic benefits deriving from early internal fixation, as well as rates of union, should be assessed. In isolated long bone fractures the survival rates to date are not so clear as those in the polytrauma cases, and there is a danger in some centres where first-class trauma facilities are available that a proportion of patients will be overtreated.

A true story may serve to illustrate this point. An anaesthetist stopped his car on a motorway in a certain European country in order to help a motor cyclist who had been involved in a road traffic accident. He quickly established that the man was not shocked, was fully conscious and had apparently suffered only a closed, minimally displaced midshaft tibial fracture. Soon after, an ambulance came along and two paramedics jumped out. They rapidly assessed the patient and one put up two intravenous infusions while the other put on an inflatable splint and gave a large dose of sedation. A few minutes later a helicopter arrived and out jumped a pretty young blonde lady in a white suit. She rushed to the patient, who was by now fairly well sedated, and following a brief physical examination, she performed a rapid anaesthetic induction. When asked why she had done this, she simply replied, 'Well, I'm an anaesthetist.'

Despite this rather interesting example of what might be called 'triage overkill', Lindsey[72] is probably correct in concluding that the teaching of the initial management of trauma should include a tendency to over-reaction rather than the opposite.

Conclusion

From the evidence in this chapter three principles clearly emerge:

1. There should be an effective triage system such as the CRAMS system to identify the patient at risk to be transferred to the appropriate hospital.

2. There is an absolute need to establish specialist trauma centres with teams representing all the relevant specialities, who are available at short notice (Figure 6.8).

3. Early internal fixation saves lives, and if used in combination with adequate vascular volume control and PEEP, the majority of trauma deaths can be prevented.

7

Fracture fixation in the elderly

G. C. Bannister, MCh Orth, FRCS, FRCS Ed Orth
A. D. Woolf, BSc, MRCP

A study of a year's fracture fixations at the Bristol Royal Infirmary, England shows that 63 per cent were carried out in patients over the age of 60 years, and 49 per cent were for proximal femoral fractures in the same age group. Proximal femoral fractures accounted for 82 per cent of all fixations in the elderly, and for 12 per cent in the under 60 age group (Figure 7.1).

The operative experience of proximal femoral fractures has long taxed the skill of the trauma surgeon, and provides the most representative model of fracture fixation in the elderly.

The aim of any fixation is stabilization of the fracture in order to rehabilitate the patient. Fracture stabilization depends on bone quality as much as the mechanical measures available to maintain stability during bone repair.

Epidemiology

Proximal femoral fractures are an enormous problem. Approximately 25 per cent of British National Health Service orthopaedic beds are occupied by patients suffering from this condition. It is the fourth commonest cause of bed occupancy within the National Health Service. Trochanteric fractures represent 60 per cent, and in Bristol fixation of this injury is the single most commonly performed orthopaedic operation.

The number of patients over 60 has increased over the last 15 years, with a concomitant rise in the incidence of fractures.

World-wide,[1] the fracture incidence is related to race, with the lowest incidence (5 in 100,000) reported from black African townships around Johannesburg. This compares with 70 cases in 100,000 in the Scandinavian countries; the rate among the Hong Kong Chinese is approximately in between. Blacks in Charlottesville, USA present with fractures at half the rate of Caucasians. Latitude does play a part as Northern European emigrants to Israel present with fractures at a lower rate than do their racial counterparts who stayed at home in a colder climate.

The female population aged over 80 exceeds the male population by 2:1, and fractures occur four times more frequently. Approximately 8 per cent of elderly females sustain a proximal femoral fracture, and 2 per cent die as a result.

Bone strength

The incidence of fractures of the hip, vertebrae, distal forearm, proximal humerus and pelvis increases with age. Why are the elderly more susceptible? Trauma is not the sole cause, as the young are more often exposed to this; rather it is the capacity of bone to resist stress. It has long been known that the elderly have thin bones and Astley Cooper, in 1824, proposed this factor as being the cause of such fractures. Decreased bone mass, coupled with increased

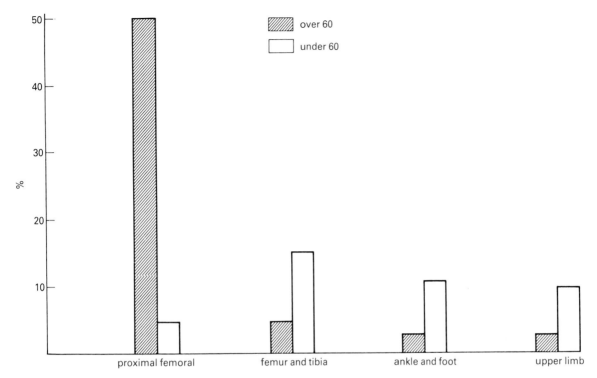

Figure 7.1 The relative proportion of fracture fixations at
Bristol Royal Infirmary, 1985–6.

porosity but normal mineralization, was termed
'osteoporosis' by the nineteenth-century pathologists,
so as to distinguish it from osteomalacia, common at
the time, in which mineral content, strength and
mineralization are reduced. Both conditions appear
as rarefied bone (osteopenia) on plain radiographs,
and both are associated with fracture.

Osteomalacia

Osteomalacia has been said to occur in up to one-
third of fractures of the proximal femur,[2] but this was
a gross overestimate, only 3 per cent being truly
osteomalacic.[3] Assessment depends on diagnostic
criteria. The elderly often have reduced serum
1,25-dihydroxy-vitamin D levels, owing to lack of
exposure to sunlight or impaired renal conversion of
25-hydroxy-vitamin D to the active metabolite. However, this does not suffice in diagnosing osteomalacia:
reduced levels of vitamin D may be adequate for

calcium absorption and bone mineralization in the
elderly. Osteomalacia can be diagnosed only by
demonstrating impairment of mineralization on histology. Widened osteoid seams are characteristic, but
these can be found in rapid bone turnover due to
other causes, and a reduction in calcification fronts is
pathognomonic. This is best demonstrated in an iliac
crest biopsy, after tetracycline labelling. The patient is
given oxytetracycline 250 mg t.d.s. for three days
before the biopsy is taken. Oxytetracycline is deposited at the calcification front, and is readily seen
under fluorescence microscopy.

A low serum calcium and elevated alkaline phosphatase are usually present in osteomalacia. These
changes are not specific enough for diagnosis, but
may prove useful in identifying which patients should
be biopsied.[3] Osteomalacia arises owing to poor diet
or lack of exposure to sunlight. Early diagnosis is
important, as the condition responds readily to treatment with vitamin D supplementation.

Osteoporosis

Age-related changes in bone mass

With age, loss of bone mass is universal in both sexes and all races. There is a high correlation between bone mineral content and bone strength in in vitro studies.[4] Various techniques have been developed to assess bone mass and its mineral content. Age-related mineral bone changes are studied on the assumption that they reflect changes in bone strength. Research has been carried out which involves measurement in large numbers of people of various ages at a single point in time. However, it assumes, perhaps incorrectly, that all individuals behave similarly regardless of prevailing dietary, social and work factors.

Bone growth reaches a peak in the third decade, following which there is a period of consolidation with decreasing cortical porosity and increased cortical thickness. Bone mass reaches a peak at around 35 years of age and then declines. Although all individuals lose bone, women are more susceptible near the menopause. This effect of hormone withdrawal is clearly demonstrated by the predictable and rapid loss of bone mass that follows oophorectomy. By the time they reach old age, women may have lost 35 per cent of cortical and 50 per cent of trabecular bone. In men, bone mass is also lost with age, but in all age groups this loss is less compared to women.

Simple osteoporosis is defined as bone mass falling below two standard deviations from the individual's expected peak bone mass; in accelerated osteoporosis, bone mass is below two standard deviations from the mean of age- and sex-matched controls.

Bone is lost all over the skeleton. However, onset, rate and amount of loss vary in cortical and trabecular bone between the axial and appendicular skeleton.[5] Cortical bone mass, estimated in the appendicular skeleton in the forearm or hand, begins to fall from the age of 40 in both men and women by 3 to 5 per cent per decade, with a superimposed phase of accelerated loss in women in the decade following the expected age of menopause.[6]

Trabecular bone forms a minority of the skeleton in terms of mass, but is metabolically most active and accounts for a larger proportion of bone turnover: annually, 60 per cent in iliac crest trabecular bone, 30 per cent in vertebral trabecular bone, compared to 3 per cent in cortical bone. In the axial skeleton, trabecular mass begins to reduce from the age of 30 to 35 years and at 6 to 8 per cent per decade in both sexes.

The entire skeleton consists of 80 per cent cortical and 20 per cent trabecular bone, but these proportions vary at different sites. Differences in the rate and timing of cortical and trabecular bone loss have been

proposed by Riggs et al, to determine the patterns of fractures seen with age.[7]

Determinants of bone mass

Bone is continually remodelling. Its mass, at any age following skeletal maturity, is a result of the peak mass attained and subsequent loss. A high life-long calcium intake is associated with a higher bone mass,[8] as are parity, frequency of lactation and oral contraceptives. Athletes have a higher bone mass, and loss of bone with disuse is well recognized.

Bone turnover occurs in discrete packets, called bone modelling units (BMU) in a cycle of osteoclastic resorption followed by osteoblastic formation lasting several months. Activation of these units determines the rate of bone turnover. In young adults, the net bone mass remains constant. With age there is impairment of bone formation in both sexes, but the rapid loss of bone mass following menopause is due to excessive resorption resulting from lack of the modulatory actions of oestrogens on bone-resorbing hormones.[9] The longer the imbalance of formation and resorption, the greater the loss of bone mass. Thus, a premature natural or surgical menopause is a major risk factor leading to a low bone mass in later life. Other factors include low body weight, smoking and alcohol. Body weight may relate to the conversion of adrenal androstenedione to oestrone in adipose tissue in postmenopausal women.

Because of a deficient diet and relative malabsorption of calcium, calcium intake in the elderly frequently falls below the levels estimated as necessary in maintaining a balance. Physical activity also plays a role and, although it falls with age, modest exercise programmes in the elderly appear to reduce the rate of bone loss.

Assessment of bone mass, mineral content and quality

Most in vitro assessments measure bone quantity and interpret this as strength. Plain radiographs are insensitive, as 30 per cent of bone mass is lost before changes become apparent. Therefore, other methods have been developed.

Changes in the shape of vertebrae, thickness of the calcar femorale or the trabecular pattern of the proximal femur (Singh index) are indicative. Although relatively crude, these assessments are simple to apply, requiring only plain radiographs, and reflect the structure in addition to mineral content.

Other methods predominantly assess mineral content. The total calcium content of the skeleton can be measured by neutron activation analysis, but costly instrumentation has limited its application to a few centres.

The appendicular skeleton is readily accessible, and simple methods of measurement exist. Metacarpal radiogrammetry, in which the cortex at midpoint of the second metacarpal is measured, is simple and inexpensive. However, it does not reflect changes in cortical porosity, a feature of aging.

Single photon absorptiometry uses the attenuation of a photon beam to measure skeletal mineral content; this is usually performed at the forearm, as the midradius consists almost entirely of cortical bone but the most distal radius and ulna contain up to 70 per cent trabecular bone. Although appendicular bone mass correlates with that in the predominantly trabecular axial skeleton, this is inadequate to predict changes from one site to another and makes direct assessment necessary.

Trabecular bone volume can be measured in the iliac crest by histomorphometric analysis of bone biopsies, but there is a large sampling error and changes at this site may not closely relate to the condition of the proximal femur or vertebral bodies.

The newer methods of dual photon absorptiometry and single energy quantitative computerized tomography are precise enough for meaningful longitudinal studies, and allow assessment of the axial skeleton at the relevant sites of the proximal femur and vertebrae. The former method measures calcium in the spinous processes and aorta, while the latter measures the marrow fat which increases with age. Dual energy computerized tomography is most precise but not readily available. These methods are expensive and time-consuming.

It may be a basic mechanical fallacy to interpret bone quantity as strength. Bone strength depends as much on its structure as on its constituent material, and most methods fail to take this into consideration.

Elderly patients with a fractured proximal femur have a significantly lower bone mass than younger healthy controls.[10] However, when fracture cases are compared to age- and sex-matched controls, the distinction is less clear.[11] Those who fracture the proximal femur do not have manifestly less bone at other sites than do age- and sex-matched controls.[11] Bone mass of the femoral neck in the non-fractured hip is less than in controls of a similar age when assessed by dual photon absorptiometry, calcar width or Singh index, but these differences are small and patients are often still within the normal range for their age. The methods cannot distinguish those who are prone to fractures from those who are not, and does not assist in identifying the small group of adults who would benefit from prophylactic treatment.

Mechanical fixation and fracture healing

Displaced intracapsular fractures

The displaced subcapital fracture remains a challenge to the surgeon. In 1935, Speed[12] recorded that, one hundred years previously, hospital museums in Europe could muster only 19 healed specimens among them. Phemister[13] recorded 76 per cent non-union and 65 per cent avascular necrosis as typical of the results of closed treatment.

The concept of impaction and fixation was proposed by Hey Groves in 1916, and was put into practice by Smith-Petersen[14] in 1931, when he introduced the trifin nail to reduce shearing at the fracture site. He achieved 75 per cent union and 15 per cent avascular necrosis.

The appearance of successive fixation devices is evidence of dissatisfaction with results. Fractures underwent bone resorption and shortened. There was confusion as to whether non-union or avascular necrosis was the major problem.

New implants emerged in an effort to overcome these complications. Goody-Moreira[15] and Pugh[16] heralded sliding screws and nails to incorporate collapse. Charnley added a spring to keep the fracture permanently under pressure. Garden considered avascular necrosis to be the major problem, and aimed for rigidity using two cannulated screws that gripped both proximal and distal fragments to maintain reduction. Results were largely comparable. The MRC prospective study of displaced subcapital fractures clarified many of the issues.[17] Union took more than six months, eventually occurred in 67 per cent of cases, and dropped from 75 per cent in the under 65 patient group to 52 per cent in the over 85. In those under 75 years of age, the Smith-Peterson nail was associated with lower union rates than was the sliding screw or crossed screws. In those over 75 years of age, the trifin nail and crossed screws were inferior to sliding implants. Delaying operation for more than three days from the time of injury resulted in higher mortality and lower rate of union.

In 1951, Moore[18] introduced his self-locking prosthesis and was followed shortly by Thompson. However, the uncemented Moore prosthesis frequently migrated within the femoral canal. This occurred four times as often as in the cemented Thompson; both prostheses caused acetabular erosion in patients under the age of 80 and in rheumatoids. Approximately 20 per cent of patients sustained complications directly related to the procedure. The best results reported 80 per cent success. In retrospective comparisons, mortality appeared higher than mortality from internal fixation.

Acetabular erosion of 10 per cent was the reported average (Figure 7.2), but this increased with time. Maxted and Denham[19] found that, after four years, over 20 per cent of cases had required further surgery to correct this. By that time, total hip replacement had become sufficiently familiar to merit consideration. However, the results from femoral neck fractures were markedly inferior to those from arthritis. Sim and Staubber[20] reported 12 per cent dislocation and 42 per cent complications; 81 per cent of patients were free of pain at the conclusion of treatment and 21 per cent died.

Acetabular erosion in younger patients was associated with excessive neck length and incongruity of prosthetic fit. A generation of biarticular hip prostheses evolved, with a greater range of head size. Early results suggested lower rates of acetabular erosion; however, the role of the joint in these prostheses was questionable, as between a quarter and a third did not demonstrate movement on radiographic screening.

The debate over internal fixation and primary prosthetic replacement was answered in principle by three randomized, prospective comparisons of the techniques (Table 7.1).[21–23] The studies drew comparable conclusions and demonstrated that primary prosthetic replacements incurred fewer reoperations, more satisfactory functional results and similar mortality within a period of six months to two years in patients over 70 years of age. Therefore, internal fixation would appear to be of value only if there are methods to improve union rates. Perosseous venography[24] and vital dyes[25] identify live heads which have significantly higher union rates (Table 7.2). The standard of reduction is equally important. Accurate reduction gave 74 per cent union compared with 44 per cent in cases of 20 degrees' malalignment. The Flynn[26] manoeuvre significantly improves the standard of closed reduction.

Figure 7.2 Acetabular erosion.

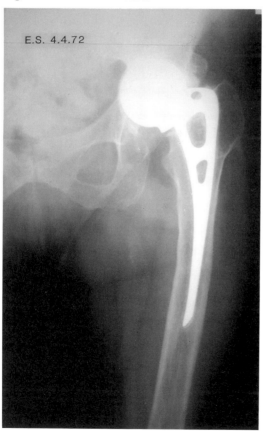

E.S. 4.4.72

Undisplaced intracapsular fractures

The only debate concerning the management of this fracture is whether or not to fix it internally. In the MRC trial, union occurred in all such fractures, and this reflects the general experience. However, Bentley[27] reported 12 per cent non-union in conservatively treated fractures, compared with 100 per cent union in those prophylactically fixed. The consequence of fixation was a slightly higher incidence of avascular necrosis, but this could be avoided if the implant was placed centrally.

Trochanteric fractures

By contrast to displaced intracapsular fractures, trochanteric fractures unite in 98 per cent of cases. Traditional management by traction for 10 to 12 weeks permitted an acceptable malunion, and internal fixation devices developed in the 1930s were aimed at accelerating mobility and reducing hospital aftercare. Fracture fixation developed for social rather than biological reasons.

Implants were developed by adding a plate to Smith-Petersen's trifin nail, and the one-piece Jewett, presented in 1941, satisfied most requirements for 40 years.

In 1949, fractures were classified as stable or

Table 7.1 Summary of randomized prospective comparisons of internal fixation and prosthetic replacement

	Implant	*Number of cases*	*Reoperation rate*	*Satisfactory (pain free)*
Soreide	Bahr screws	51	18	71
	Christiansen prosthesis	53	6	92
Riley	Cross screws	66	8.5	63
	Moore or Thompson prosthesis	85	9	83
Sikorski	Garden screws	104	38	40
	Thompson prosthesis	114	9	76

Table 7.2 Union rates of live and dead heads (per cent)

	Technique	*Viable*	*Non-viable*	*Ratio*
Outerbridge	Perosseous venography	88	47	1.87
Milligan	Kiton Green	83	38	2.1

unstable by Evans[28] (Figure 7.3). Although his description related to fracture behaviour on traction, it carries the most accurate prediction of fracture behaviour following internal fixation. The problem with all classifications is their limited accuracy, as a proportion of those predicted to remain stable subsequently displace.

The natural tendency of the trochanteric fracture is to fill the void caused by medial comminution and to unite in varus. The proportion of three-part fractures has risen since Evans's report.

Three families of implants have been employed to hold trochanteric fractures: fixed length nail plates, sliding nail plates and condylocephalic nails.

The fixed length nail plate was shown to secure union but penetrated the acetabulum (Figure 7.4) and bent or broke in over half the comminuted fractures. These complications were more irritating than catastrophic. The nail usually penetrated the head medial to the weight-bearing surface. A bent nail was harmless to the patient whose fracture united, and if an implant broke, fracture union usually occurred after a short period of traction. However, a proportion of patients had to undergo further surgery because of implant failure, and the subject invited further study. Even impacted fractures demand that the implant bears 25 per cent of body weight (or 75 lb). Some of the earlier implants barely met these demands. In 1954, Holt[29] subjected existing nail plates to stress testing; he noted failure of the Thornton and Neufeld devices at 60 lb, and failure of the Jewett device at 140 lb. As a result, Holt designed a device which bolted the plate to the femoral shaft and was capable of withstanding 840 lb, with a reduced incidence of implant fracture but no overall improvement.

Sarmiento and Williams[30] noted that the strength of an implant could be improved by increasing its nail plate angle. This produced a gain of 6 per cent for every 5 degrees of valgus, but the nail inevitably embedded in the upper outer quadrant of the head and cut out.

Intramedullary methylmethacrylate support for a nail plate did not appear to reduce union (97 per cent). This technique remains of value in malignancy or for patients with an anticipated short lifespan.

Limitations of the fixed length nail plate resulted in approximately one reoperation for every six cases of acetabular penetration, and it was against this background that surgeons turned to the sliding screw devices in the 1960s. These implants were devised to improve union of subcapital fractures (see above) but results in trochanteric fractures were more encouraging. The Seattle experience showed reduction of mechanical failure to 1 per cent.[31]

Uncontrolled comparisons with fixed length nail plates suggested that mechanical failure and reoperation could be reduced up to five times by using sliding screws (Figure 7.5). This seems to be

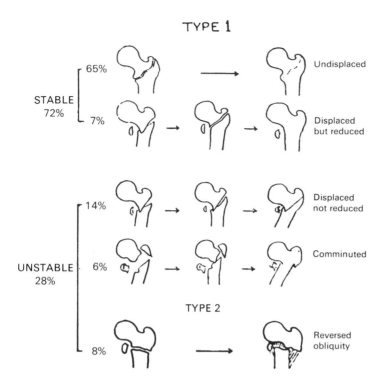

Figure 7.3 The classification of trochanteric fractures.

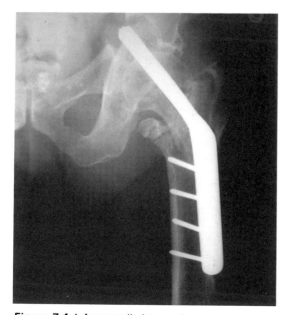

Figure 7.4 A Jewett nail plate eroding an acetabulum.

confirmed by results emerging from controlled trials, for three reasons: first, the devices are strong; second, they grip the proximal fragment; third, they collapse, allowing more weight-bearing by the bone. The optimum resolution of forces for the sliding screws is 160 degrees, and the 135 degrees' implant slides less well. The four-part fractures that impact best comprise only 10 per cent of the total, and in the three-part lesions a tendency to varus displacement puts the screw under tension. None the less, the sliding screws represent an advance over fixed length nail plates, as their strength and proximal grip are important in most fractures.

Osteotomy to establish continuity of medial bone is a logical adjunct to fixation devices that inevitably break if they hold the fracture distracted.[32] Sarmiento's valgus osteotomies reduced mechanical complication to 5 per cent in an initial report, but controlled trials failed to demonstrate significant advantage over a Jewett nail plate in an aligned reduction.

The medial displacement osteotomy in the hands of Dimon and Hughston reduced complications in comminuted fractures, but the same results were not reproduced by others. Hunter[33] found this procedure actually to increase complications.

Interpretation of data

The mechanical results of treatment have changed very little. For example, Smith-Petersen's union rates for displaced subcapital fractures have been exceeded only sporadically. Equally, trochanteric fractures do not unite more frequently with modern fixation devices than they did in the past, although occupancy of hospital beds has decreased considerably.

Most of the research on this topic has been in the form of retrospective audit in a particular situation. However, such localized results provide no information as to what is likely to recur under similar circumstances elsewhere. A randomized, prospective controlled trial is required to establish this type of information. Such studies are very demanding and more glibly suggested than undertaken, but if properly conducted they provide a considerably higher level of information than potentially misleading audits.

A case to consider is the experience of Bath Hospital with Enders nails, reported in 1981: a retrospective comparison of these nails (Figure 7.6) with a variety

of nail plate fixation strongly favoured the condylocephalic nails. Reoperation and severe malunion were reported in 2 and 12 per cent of cases respectively, and two years later[34] 14 per cent reoperation and 80 per cent malunion were the result of this change of policy.

In the burgeoning face of new fixation devices for displaced subcapital fractures, the MRC prospective trial failed to reproduce significant differences among all but the original trifin nail, and a controlled trial by McQuillan et al[35] has demonstrated that two of these nails are superior to one.

The posterior approach to the hip for Thompson hemiarthroplasty was shown to result in more infections, dislocations and higher mortality at Bath Hospital. Yet a controlled trial in Bristol only 10 miles away showed higher infection rates from the anterior approach and equal numbers of dislocation from both approaches, and reproduced only the associated mortality rates.

Mortality has been shown to vary among hospitals within the same city.[30,31] In Bristol, three-month mortality from trochanteric fractures rose from 17 per cent in 1974–6 to 31 per cent in 1981–2. Retrospective claims arising from comparisons of varying material between different centres and hospitals at different times must be viewed with extreme circumspection.

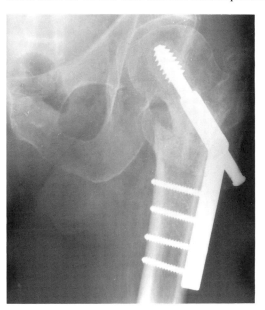

Figure 7.5 The sliding screw device for trochanteric fracture.

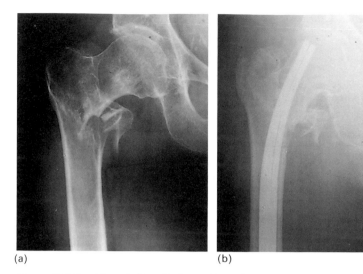

(a)   (b)   (c)

Figure 7.6 Condylocephalic nails for trochanteric fracture: *a*, original fracture; *b*, post operation; *c*, appearance at 6 weeks.

Rehabilitation

The choice of fixation depends on the patient's degree of activity and life expectancy. If the surgeon could predict a patient's longevity, total hip replacement instead of a hemiarthroplasty might be performed, to prevent additional surgery in old age. Likewise, if the surgeon were to know in advance whether a patient was likely to return home after surgery, arrangements for social support or sheltered accommodation could be made; and if the physiotherapist were to know which patients would walk again regardless, which would be permanently bedridden and which would benefit from special programmes, efforts could be directed accordingly.

To some extent, such predictions can be made. Mortality has been studied frequently (Table 7.3).[36] In most series, two-thirds of patients are living at home and a third come from sheltered accommodation or institutions. Those living at home have four times as great a chance of survival as the average, and those who are institutionalized have only half the mean rate. Injury outside the home is consistent with independence and was observed in the Newcastle data but was not sought elsewhere. A low score in Roth's mental test, or an age exceeding 85 years, increase the chances of mortality.[37] Thus, an 80-year-old institutionalized patient with no caring relatives carries a 16 per cent chance of surviving a proximal femoral fracture if the unit survival rate was 75 per cent.[38]

Morbidity has been less extensively studied.[39] How-

Table 7.3 Factors affecting survival

Criterion	Ratio
Total independence	4
Injury in a public place	2.5
Hospital	2
Caring relative	1.5
Low mental test score	0.6
Age less than 85	0.6
Total dependence	0.6

ever, if the patients live in their own homes, their chances of returning are 2.6 times higher for those under 75 years of age. This rate is higher if they do not have a medical disorder that hinders their rehabilitation, if they have someone living with them, and if they can walk with a frame within two weeks of the time of fracture. A combination of these three factors provides an accurate assessment of rehabilitation potential (Table 7.4).

The patient's ultimate mobility has not been extensively studied. The findings at the Bristol Royal Infirmary (Table 7.5) showed that 30 to 50 per cent of patients regained their original mobility and a further 20 per cent dropped by one grade, requiring a walking stick or a frame. Mobility improved in 7 per cent of cases. Independence at home before injury suggested a chance of mobility (with a walking stick) three times

Table 7.4 Factors affecting return to own home

	Ratio
Age under 75	2.6
Absence of medical condition affecting rehabilitation	1.3
Living with someone	1.3
Walking with a frame	1.1

greater than in patients who needed a walking aid before injury. Relative youth (under 75 years) before injury, capacity to walk a quarter of a mile and ability to walk unaided were all positive indications of good recovery.

The majority of the above factors *cannot be influenced by orthopaedic surgeons*. Old age, the break-up of the extended family, the ravages of Alzheimer's disease and atherosclerosis are adverse factors in effective rehabilitation after fracture stabilization.

Orthogeriatric units have been set up following Devas's enthusiasm and interest in the subject. To date, they have been introduced in Hastings and Nottingham,[40] and reports emanating from their surgeons emphasize improvement in the occupancy rate of hospital beds, space for patients and morale. Unfortunately, there is no evidence that patients are rehabilitated better; the Hastings unit returned fewer patients to their homes than the Newcastle unit, and Nottingham's criteria for admission to the unit were left to the individual choice of a number of orthopaedic trainees. The concept is exciting, and standardization of the variables outlined in this chapter would contribute to resolving doubts about the efficacy of these units. This is vital, as hospital variables seem to be the single most promising factor that can be influenced.

After fixation and rehabilitation, prevention of further fracture must be considered.

Table 7.5 Factors affecting final mobility

	Ratio
Independence in own home before fracture	3
Under 75	2.6
Walking 0.25 mile	1.5
Walking unaided	1.3

Prevention of bone disorders

Elderly patients sustaining a fracture of the proximal femur are at risk of other age-related fractures. They will already have a low bone mass, which puts them at risk of fracture at this and other sites following a sufficiently serious fall. Of Danish women over the age of 75, 85 per cent with vertebral fractures had sustained at least one other type of fracture,[41] and vertebral deformity or compression fractures in routine chest radiographs are twice as common in patients with hip and Colles fractures as in age-matched controls.[42]

To date, there is no treatment providing a long-lasting restoration of lost bone mass; and even if bone mass could indeed be restored it would have to be deposited in the appropriate way in order to induce strength. Loss of trabeculae is irreversible and thickening of remaining trabeculae may have no significant effect on strength and resistance to trauma. At present, management is limited to prevention of further loss of bone mass. The age of the patient also limits the scope of treatment, as it may take several years to alter bone mass significantly.

Any treatment of osteoporosis must be capable of reducing the risk of fracture, and long-term studies on a large number of patients are needed to show a significant effect. Such studies have not been carried out. Many therapeutic trials have used changes in bone mass as an outcome measure, assessed at various sites, many of which have little relevance to the risk of fracture at the proximal femur.

Calcium

Calcium is deficient in the osteoporotic bone, and is poorly absorbed in old age. The average calcium intake that achieves neutral balance is 1500 mg per day in oestrogen-deprived women, but actual intake is close to 500 mg per day.[43] It would seem logical, although simplistic, that to reverse this negative calcium balance would restore bone mass. It is known that a high calcium intake increases peak bone mass,[8] but the effects of calcium supplementation on subsequent bone loss are disputed. Some studies have shown a reduction in bone loss from cortical sites,[44,45] but other trials have found calcium supplementation to be ineffective.[46] There is a lack of data on the effect of calcium supplementation on femoral neck mass or the incidence of proximal femur fracture.

Despite the conflicting evidence, a recent NIH Consensus Conference recommended a daily calcium intake of 1000–1500 mg, in the diet or with tablet supplements, in an attempt to suppress age-related bone loss and reduce the fracture rate associated with osteoporosis.[47]

Hormone replacement therapy

Hormone replacement therapy is the only treatment to prevent loss of bone mass and inhibit bone resorption, if it is started within three years following menopause. After eight to ten years the effectiveness of this therapy is reduced, possibly because non-hormone-dependent bone loss (senile osteoporosis) comes into play. Case-control studies have shown that long-term oestrogen treatment, started at or near the age of menopause, results in reduction of fracture rates, including those of the proximal femur.[42,48] However, there is little evidence of the effects of treatment on established osteoporosis, especially as such patients tend to be around or over 75 years of age.

Continuous oestrogens are associated with an increased risk of endometrial cancer,[49] but if given in combination with progestogens for 12 days this risk is eliminated,[50] perhaps with a protective effect against endometrial carcinoma. They may even show a positive action against ischaemic heart disease; the natural oestrogens present no risk of thromboembolic disease.

Fluoride

Fluoride is an effective stimulator of bone formation and will have a complementary effect if used in combination with oestrogens, as has been demonstrated by the marked reduction of vertebral fracture rates.[51] It induces excessive osteoid, which is preventable in most cases by the addition of calcium. Trabecular bone mass increases, but some studies have found no change in total body calcium. This has raised the concern that fluoride is merely redistributing calcium from cortical to trabecular bone.[52]

In a partly retrospective case-control study, fluoride and calcium treatment reduced vertebral fracture rate, but it was almost abolished with the combination of calcium, fluoride and oestrogen therapy.[51] The results of two long-term controlled trials are awaited and many still consider fluoride therapy to be experimental. It certainly produces frequent adverse effects, with up to 50 per cent experiencing rheumatic and gastrointestinal symptoms. This is not surprising, as some hydrofluoric acid will form in the stomach.

The promise of fluoride has been tempered by gastrointestinal side-effects and at present continuing hormone therapy and a diet high in calcium offer the best chance of prevention of bone disease; but it will be some time before the beneficial effect of this treatment is established. If the concept of a fracture threshold is correct a small improvement of true bone strength could postpone a fracture until the tenth decade, by which time the susceptible population will have declined from other causes.

8

The Herbert bone screw and osteochondral fractures

T. D. Scott, BSc, MB, ChB, FRCS,
FRCS Ed Orth
T. D. Bunker, BSc, MB, BS, MCh Orth,
FRCS, FRCS Ed

Displaced intra-articular fractures remain a fascinating challenge to the trauma surgeon. Hippocrates wrote that cartilage did not 'heal and join together again'. Thus, severely displaced intra-articular fractures may lead to deformity, often with accompanying stiffness and pain.

It is not surprising, therefore, that the earliest attempts at both internal and external fixation were for displaced intra-articular fractures; in 1883, Lister internally fixed an olecranon gap fracture[1] with a wire loop, and in 1834 Malgaigne used his external fixation clamp to hold a patellar gap fracture.[2]

Internal fixation was revitalized by the Swiss AO/ASIF group as a method of preventing joint stiffness by anatomical reduction and rigid fixation of the fracture, followed by early joint movement. Although first used in diaphyseal fractures, these principles were soon applied to intra-articular fractures. As the 'tool boxes' increased in size, implants decreased in size and surgeons' experience improved, so more and more difficult intra-articular fractures could be tackled.

Satisfactory fixation of small osteochondral fractures remained technically difficult. If not vital for joint stability or function, these small fragments may be left or excised and the defect allowed to fill with fibrocartilage. Sometimes, however, they can be vital to joint function (Figure 8.1: two-thirds of the femoral head, representing the major weight-bearing surface, was sheared off in this 22 year old man). Even when countersunk, the smallest AO screws would, in this situation, leave a head protruding (Figure 8.2), which is bound to score the opposing articular surface.

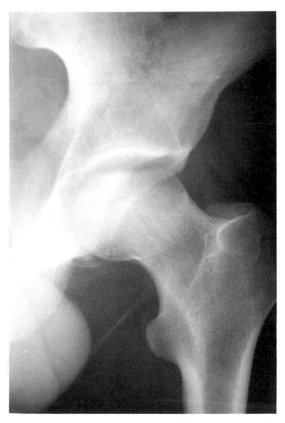

Figure 8.1 Osteochondral fracture of the femoral head.

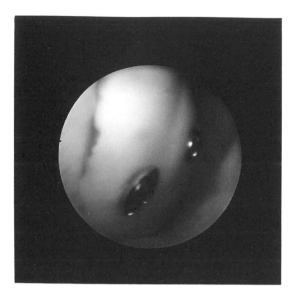

Figure 8.2 The head of a normal bone screw protrudes into the joint.

Kirschner wires have been used to fix small fragments such as displaced radial head fractures,[3,4] and although good results have been reported, they tend not only to back out, scoring the opposing articular cartilage, but also to migrate inside the body. Kirschner wires cannot cause rigid fixation or compression, owing to their smooth nature.

The Herbert differential pitch bone screw was designed by Herbert and Fisher[5] for internal fixation of scaphoid fractures (a truly intra-articular fracture), as a result of their dissatisfaction with Kirschner wires and cancellous lag screws. This entirely new concept in screw fixation has a second thread in place of the normal screw head, allowing the implant to be totally buried within the bone. The screw can be inserted through articular cartilage, causing very little damage; the head then virtually disappears (Figure 8.3). The differential pitch of leading and trailing screw threads means that compression is then applied across the fracture site. As well as the screw, Herbert and Fisher developed a jig through which drilling, tapping and screw insertion could be performed, while it held the fracture reduced.

The differential pitch bone screw is the technical solution to the fixation of many osteochondral fractures,[6–8] and the authors have used it in over 100 patients. In this chapter, its use, advantages and disadvantages in the hand, wrist, elbow, hip, knee and ankle will be discussed. First, however, the normal morphology of hyaline articular cartilage and its response to blunt, superficial and deep trauma, as well as cartilage repair, should be considered.

Morphology

Normal hyaline articular cartilage consists of a uniform matrix in which isolated chondrocytes are scattered; there are no blood vessels, lymphatics or nerve fibres. The chondrocytes occupy less than 1 per cent by volume of the cartilage. The rest is matrix.

The matrix is 70 per cent to 80 per cent water; half the dry mass is composed of collagen and half of glycoprotein. The collagen is unique to articular cartilage (Type II), and characterized by three α_1 chains in a triple helix configuration. The fibrils are finer than those of tendon, skin and bone (Type I). The collagen fibrils are so placed as to withstand the pressures put upon the loaded cartilage, arranged tangentially on the surface (to withstand surface tension and shearing forces), and vertically in the deeper layers (to withstand compressive forces). Benninghoff,[9] in 1925, proposed that the collagen fibres must be orientated in arcades from the subchondral bone plate to the surface and back (Figure 8.4). MacConnail[10] suggested that a more oblique orientation, filled in with a random mesh, would resist

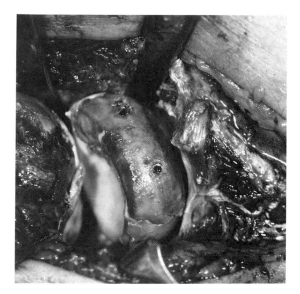

Figure 8.3 The head of the Herbert screw disappears under the cartilage.

loads better within cartilage as the contact area shifted, but this theory was not substantiated by scanning electron microscopy, which tended to support Benninghoff's theory. Broom[11] has tried to combine both the need for a random mesh and the factual

evidence in favour of Benninghoff's arcades by proposing that the arcades coil around each other as they ascend and descend, allowing tangential surface and deeper vertical orientation.

Trapped within the cartilage fibres, mainly in the central random mesh area, lie the proteoglycans which in turn attract water. The proteoglycans are enormous molecules with a molecular weight of 1 to 2 million. They are composed of a protein core with side chains of chondroitin 4, chondroitin 6 and keratin sulphate. There is more keratin sulphate in the deeper layers and in the elderly. These enormous molecules are linked at one end to a long thread-like molecule of hyaluronic acid, the link being stabilized by a link protein (Figure 8.5). The entire mass sucks water in to form a firm jelly caught in the random mesh of collagen fibrils.

Just next to the subchondral bone plate the cartilage becomes calcified, and the boundary between the deep calcified layer and the remaining cartilage is called the 'tidemark': a 2 to 5μ thick, undulating layer of collagen fibres running parallel to the subchondral bone plate (Figure 8.6). The calcified layer is usually 0.1 mm thick, and the hyaline cartilage above it varies in thickness in human joints, being 0.03 mm to 4 mm thick.

The chondrocytes vary in size, shape and distribution, being flatter, smaller and more closely packed in the superficial layer, uniformly distributed in the intermediate layer and arranged in a columnar fashion in the deeper layers. Despite the fact that no chondrocyte replication has been demonstrated in

Figure 8.4 *a* Benninghoff's arcades, *b* MacConnail's random mesh and *c* Bloom's mixture.

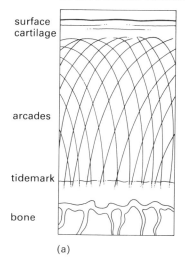

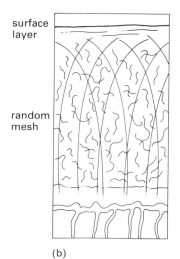

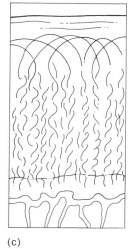

(a) (b) (c)

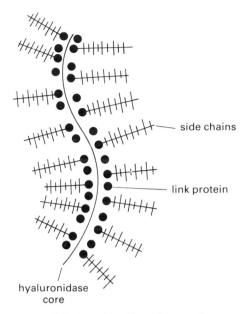

side chains

link protein

hyaluronidase
core

Figure 8.5 The composition of proteoglycan.

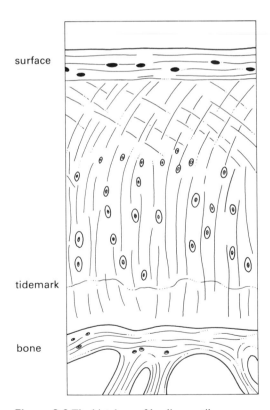

surface

tidemark

bone

Figure 8.6 The histology of hyaline cartilage.

adult articular cartilage,[12,13] synthesis of collagen and proteoglycan has been demonstrated by radiolabelling techniques. Chondrocytes are just as active as any other cell in the body, and the lack of replication is due only to there being very few of them. Proteoglycan turnover occurs in two parts: the faster part in 45 days and the slower in 250–500 days. Turnover time for collagen is about 300 years.

In immature joints, small blood vessels perforate the bony end plates entering the calcified layer. In adults, the subchondral bone becomes solid,[14] so that chondrocyte nutrition is totally dependent upon diffusion of metabolites from synovial fluid through the matrix. Alterations in the matrix affect this diffusion, as does the composition of synovial fluid and its circulation.

Electrolytes, water, amino acids and glucose diffuse freely inside the cartilage matrix. Joint movement appears to be essential to cartilage nutrition, as movement and cyclical loading pump small molecules through the cartilage matrix. However, if a joint is immobilized, a stagnant film of synovial fluid forms over the surface of the cartilage, diffusion slows down and the deeper chondrocytes are at risk.

Chondrocyte metabolism is also affected by general factors, such as variation in oxygen tension,[15] pH,[16] calcium concentration[17] and cortisol.[18]

All the enzymes known to degrade proteoglycans have been identified in articular cartilage, except hyaluronidase which is present in synovial membrane. Inhibitors of proteolytic activity have also been extracted from articular cartilage.

Response to blunt injury

Cartilage often sustains direct injury without an articular fracture occurring. For instance, in a dashboard injury causing a fracture of the femur, massive compressive loads are transmitted via the articular cartilage of the knee to the femur which then explodes. Obviously, these forces are likely to damage the articular cartilage of the knee and hip. The amount of damage sustained depends on the surface area of the joint that absorbs the load, the size of the load and the velocity with which that load is applied.

Repo and Finlay[19] performed a series of elegant experiments on live human tibial plateau articular cartilage to determine the nature and extent of these injuries. The tibial plateaux were harvested from transplant donors and stored in culture medium; the experiments were performed within twelve hours of harvesting. It was found that there was a critical stress limit, beyond which articular cartilage sustained damage in increasing proportion to the violence expended upon it. The critical limit appeared to be 25

Newtons/mm². The average peak stress on the tibial plateau during walking is about 4 Newtons/mm². The compressive force necessary to fracture a femur is in the range 7 to 12 K Newtons, and it may be deduced that the critical limit for the average size hip is 9 K Newtons; therefore, this amount of force is capable of causing significant cartilage damage.

What is the cartilage damage? Repo and Finlay assessed it by scanning electron microscopy, and cell viability was determined by tritiated proline uptake. Their studies showed that cartilage stressed beyond the critical limit started to fissure, with cell death in the surface zone and alongside the fissures. As the stress increased, so did the extent of fissuring, both major (from the surface to the subchondral plate) and minor (surface only). In the most damaged group, where there was extensive maceration and fissuring, only the basal chondrocytes demonstrated consistent proline uptake.

Partial thickness injury

The controversy over whether articular cartilage lacerations heal started with John Hunter's in vivo experiments. Redfern, in the 1850s, performed a series of experiments on live dogs and concluded, 'I no longer entertain the slightest doubt that wounds in articular cartilage are capable of perfect union by formation of fibrous tissue out of the texture of the cut surfaces.'

Articular cartilage scarification was used by Meachim[20] to study healing of partial thickness defects. He, like Redfern, showed proliferation of chondrocytes adjacent to the injury. However, these cells do not appear to be producing Type II collagen in sufficient quantities to affect repair with hyaline cartilage. Superficial fibroblasts appear to fill in the defect with fibrocartilage.[21]

In the longer term, it appears that these superficial lacerations stabilize and do not, despite the irregularity, progress to osteoarthritis or chondromalacia.[22] Similar findings have been noted following tangential partial thickness defects.

Deep penetrating injuries

As these injuries penetrate the subchondral bone, the defect is immediately filled by blood. Thus, the whole repair is altered with invasion of fibroblasts into the enriched fibrin clot,[23] which is followed by ingrowth of capillaries producing an initial loose fibrovascular network that becomes more cellular and less vascular.

Normal bone healing occurs in the subchondral bone, but this does not extend into the calcified layer of the cartilage. The fibrous scar tissue lacks the normal orientation of collagen fibrils, particularly at the surface which tends to fibrillate, but it may function well for many years.

Repair of osteochondral fractures

In 1850, Sir James Paget wrote, 'There are, I believe, no instances in which a lost portion of cartilage has been restored, or a wounded portion repaired, with new and well-formed perfect cartilage, in the human subjects'. Little seems to have changed since his time to contradict this statement. However, there is experimental evidence of perfect healing in both mature and immature small mammals, and this has led to rigid fixation of osteochondral fractures, in an attempt to obtain perfect healing.

The experimental work of Salter et al[24] on the repair of full thickness cartilage defects and osteochondral fractures has received much criticism, as it was mostly performed on immature rabbits. Immature articular cartilage is supplied from vessels crossing the subchondral bone plate, which does not occur in the adult. In spite of this, their work is well worth reviewing.

Full thickness cartilage defects (produced by drilling rabbit knees) healed with fibrous tissue in 75 per cent of caged animals; 25 per cent healed with poorly differentiated mesenchymal tissue or hyaline cartilage, less in adults. If the rabbit knee was immobilized in plaster, there was very little sign of healing at three weeks, and at ten weeks numerous extensive intra-articular adhesions were seen in the region of the defects. This is to be expected on the basis of diffusion of cartilage nutrient being dependent on circulation of synovial fluid. Rabbits on continuous passive motion (CPM) showed not only more rapid healing, but healing with hyaline cartilage in 52 per cent of defects (slightly less in adults).

An experimental model of a Salter IV intra-articular fracture was then used, and anatomical reduction and rigid fixation with an AO screw performed. At four weeks, the range of knee movement was normal in the caged animals, but the fracture line was clearly visible in most knee joints. Eighty per cent of animals put into plaster showed grossly limited movement, and all had clearly visible fracture lines. Rabbits on CPM had a full range of movement, no adhesions, and in 80 per cent the fracture line had disappeared (Figure 8.7). Moreover, the fracture site was filled with tissue resembling hyaline cartilage.

Mitchell and Shephard[25] examined the healing of

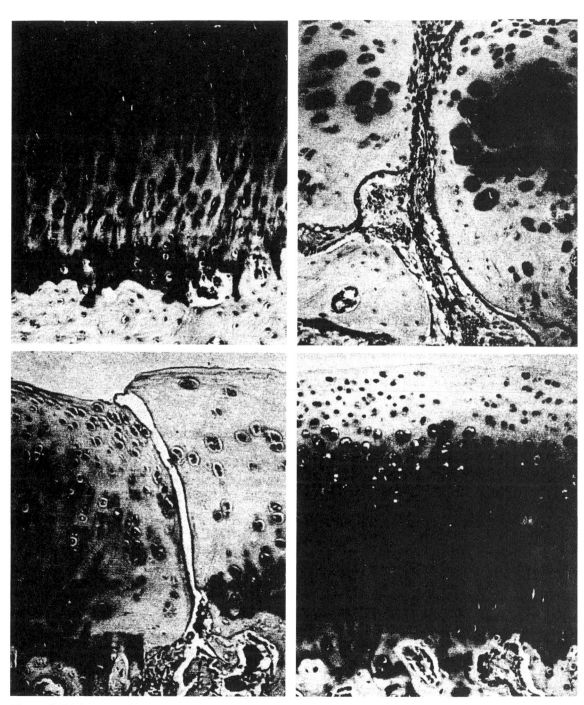

Figure 8.7 Salter's experimental findings: *top left*, normal cartilage; *top right*, immobilization—fibrous tissue fills the defect and an adhesion overlies the articular surface; *bottom left*, cage activity, persistent gap in the cartilage; *bottom right*, rigid fixation and CPM, showing cartilage healing.

intra-articular fractures in adult rabbits. Three groups were studied: incomplete reduction; adequate reduction and fixation without compression using an AO screw; and rigid fixation with compression. The results were studied at seven weeks to one year, with transmission and scanning electron microscopy.

The first two groups healed with fibrocartilage. The third, rigidly fixed, group healed with tissue which by electron microscopy appeared to be hyaline cartilage. Mitchell and Shepard felt that coaptation of the joint surfaces prevented the ingrowth of granulation tissue, or created an environment that allowed chondrocytes from the tidemark region to heal the defect with hyaline cartilage.

These experiments rationalize rigid fixation with compression of intra-articular fractures in man, followed by early joint movement. Thus, reconstruction of fractured joint surfaces becomes appealing macroscopically, microscopically and physiologically.

The hand

Fracture fixation

The Herbert screw was used to fix one Bennett fracture dislocation. Although elegant, it has no advantages over a 1.5 mm or 2.0 mm AO screw in this situation, and there are easier ways to hold a Bennett fracture reduced.

The Herbert screw has also been used for a condylar fracture of the proximal phalanx, but even the 16 mm screw stands out on either side of the joint and offers no advantages over a conventional screw. Shorter screws and a trailing thread tap are being designed.

Joint fusion

Faithful and Herbert[26] have reported their results on the arthrodesis of joints in the hand in 26 cases. The main indication was pain and deformity of the distal interphalangeal joint. All arthrodeses united, and external splintage was not necessary following surgery.

The wrist

The scaphoid fracture and its sequelae are the major indications for the use of the Herbert screw, although fractures of the trapezium and intercarpal fusions have also been reported. Many questions remain unanswered in relation to the scaphoid, for example, how should they be classifed? Do they unite? When is a scaphoid united? Does it matter? What are the indications for surgery? What approach should be used? Why should the Herbert screw be used? Some of these questions will be tackled below.

Classification

Russe[27] classified scaphoid fractures according to site (proximal, middle and distal thirds) and obliquity (horizontal, oblique, transverse and vertical oblique). Proximal third fractures were slow to unite owing to their poor blood supply, while vertical oblique fractures were slow to unite owing to their instability, which Russe compared with the Pauwels III fracture of the femoral neck.

The Mayo group[28] have preferred to classify scaphoid fractures as stable or unstable. Stable fractures have an intact periosteal hinge or incomplete damage of the cartilage. Ninety-five per cent of these united. Unstable fractures have an offset of 1 mm between the bone ends or 15 degrees of lunatoscaphoid angulation or more than 45 degrees of scapholunate angulation; in other words, detectable intercalary segment instability. Only 54 per cent of unstable fractures united.

The Herbert classification (Figure 8.8) initially appears cumbersome, but covers all eventualities. Group A are stable fractures, group B are unstable fractures and group D are non-unions. This classification is useful both prognostically and in identifying patients who would benefit from surgery.

Do scaphoids unite?

Stimson[29] stated that total disability of the wrist was the normal consequence of a scaphoid fracture, and Codman was equally pessimistic. In 1928, Adams and Leonard[30] wrote, 'It is undisputed that, in the majority of cases, the bone does not unite'. Lemerle's group[31] reported a non-union rate of 36 per cent. In 1954 came the great turnaround when Böhler's group reported a 76 per cent union rate in over 700 fractures.[32] Russe reported 97 per cent union in 220 fractures, and London[33] 95 per cent in 227 cases. Both surgeons acknowledged the great difficulty in diagnosing union, as trabeculae may appear to span the fracture in one radiographic view, yet an obvious fracture gap can be seen in another view taken on the same day. Russe took the sclerotic line to be evidence of union. However, the true significance of this line needs to be validated; Leslie and Dickson,[34] who also

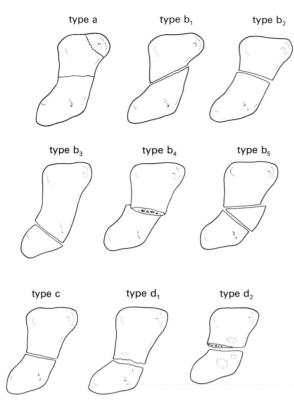

type a   type b$_1$ type b$_2$

type b$_3$ type b$_4$ type b$_5$

type c   type d$_1$ type d$_2$

Figure 8.8 The Herbert classification.

Does union matter?

Most surgeons have treated patients with minor trauma whose radiographs show a long-term sclerotic non-union; such patients may have been employed in heavy manual work for a considerable time. However, Ruby[35] showed that 97 per cent of patients presenting with a painful scaphoid non-union, at least five years following injury, have evidence of degenerative arthritis of the wrist, and that this incidence increases according to the length of time since the injury. Mack[36] showed a steady progression of arthritis in 47 patients with symptomatic non-union.

Can poor results be predicted?

London felt that poor results could not be predicted, but displacement of the fracture, and particularly progressive displacement, was a poor prognostic factor according to other authorities.[5,35] Increased lucency of the fracture gap and early cyst formation were also poor prognostic factors. Delay in diagnosis, carpal instability and fracture dislocations all carry a high risk.

These unresolved questions are of vital importance. The incidence of non-union in scaphoid fractures is second only to subcapital femoral fractures. Both are entirely intra-articular. A non-union rate of 36 to 50 per cent is not acceptable in displaced subcapital femoral fractures. Therefore why should it be acceptable in displaced scaphoid fractures? Use of the hand is arguably as vital as function of the femur, and non-union is more common in the dominant hand.[34]

The optimistic papers of Böhler, Russe and London have led to a virtually universal non-operative management of scaphoid fractures. However, the Mayo group[28] and Herbert[5] recommend internal fixation for displaced fresh fractures. Herbert goes further and states that although stable (grade A) fractures unite if kept for two or three months in plaster, working people consider this a financial strain. Herbert would recommend surgery for selected undisplaced fractures. Postoperatively, the patient should wear a removable orthoplast brace.

At present, however, only symptomatic non-union is universally an indication for surgery. It cannot be denied that too many symptomatic non-unions of the scaphoid are seen, and that they are more difficult to treat than fresh fractures. Union rates following internal fixation of scaphoid non-union with conventional lag screws vary from 16 per cent to 87 per cent.[37] This should be compared to 85 per cent union with Russe grafting in expert hands,[28,38,39] as long as the fracture is held in plaster for at least four months postoperatively. We have reported our results in 50 Herbert

took this as their radiological determinant of union, showed a consistently higher incidence of sclerotic line as a result of non-union rather than union. This calls Russe's 97 union rate into question.

London believed that radiological union was of no consequence, and wrote that many of the cases which united 'did not quite reach this unequivocal standard' of radiological union. He stated, quite rightly, that the wrist should be treated as opposed to the radiograph, but this calls into question his 95 per cent union rate.

More recently, the Mayo group[28] reported a non-union rate of 46 per cent for displaced scaphoid fractures, and Herbert[5] believes that the true incidence of union may be as low as 50 per cent. Thus, there seems to have been a cycle through the century: first great pessimism, then great optimism, and currently a more balanced view.

screw fixations,[7] with a union rate of 82 per cent for sclerotic non-union and 88 per cent for fibrous non-union.

What approach should be used?

The classic approach to the scaphoid is a bayonet radial incision through the anatomical snuff box. The authors prefer the Herbert approach, a curved 5 cm volar approach to the subcutaneous tubercle of the scaphoid via the bed of flexor carpi radialis. The palmar branch of the radial artery is often large and must be ligated. The strong radio-scaphocapitate ligament is divided, allowing a clear view of the entire scaphoid bone.

The Herbert scaphoid jig seems easy to use, but it is not. Thirteen cases of technical difficulty were recorded in our 50 cases. This reflected the fact that 17 surgeons who used the device were all relatively inexperienced. Can we learn from their errors?

The commonest technical error involved placing the screw too near the volar cortex of the scaphoid. The scaphoid axis lies at 45 degrees to the long axis of the arm (Figure 8.9), and the jig must be placed in this deep alignment. This means that the hooked tip of the jig must not be placed on the tip of the proximal pole but dropped through the radioscaphoid joint and hooked on to the dorsal surface of the scaphoid. It is difficult for surgeons accustomed to anteroposterior radiographs of the scaphoid to appreciate the scaphoid from the lateral view, but an articulated skeleton shows the vastness of the dorsal articular surface. It is into this large piece of bone that the jig must be directed. In life the scaphoid and lunate should be

Figure 8.9 *a*, The scaphoid axis lies at 45 degrees to the long axis of the arm; *b*, if the screw is inserted at a lesser angle it lies too volar.

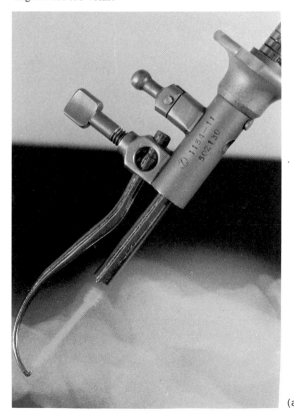

(a)

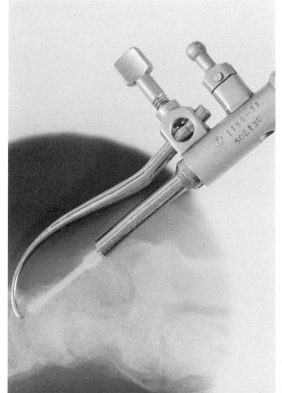

(b)

considered one, as the strong scapholunate ligament combines them into an entity; this fact is not appreciated in the study of radiographs.

Unstable fractures tend to buckle into a flexed position. Compression of the jig increases this deformity, making the procedure even more difficult. In these cases, a temporary Kirschner wire should first be placed to prevent collapse, and if the collapse is severe a wedge cancellous graft must be inserted to correct the malunion.

In the fibrous non-union group, an 88 per cent union rate was achieved by excising it and packing the defect with cancellous graft obtained with a bone biopsy trephine via a 7 mm stab incision. The two failures in this group were not grafted as they should have been.

However, in the sclerotic non-union group it is essential to resect the sclerotic ends with a sharp, fine chisel, and to insert a corticocancellous graft from the iliac crest so as to 'jack out' the malunion. With this procedure there was an 82 per cent rate of union, with three cases of failure; one patient was not grafted, one had had two previous failed Russe grafts, and in the third the screw was too short, with inadequate hold.

One fresh fracture dislocation failed to unite. This was a severely displaced and collapsed scaphoid that had not been grafted. Herbert states that these are the most technically demanding cases, and there should be no hesitation in grafting them.

The average time for a patient to return to work was 10 weeks for fresh fractures, 6.4 weeks for fibrous non-unions and 11.2 weeks for sclerotic non-unions.

Herbert and Fischer,[5] in 158 procedures, showed 100 per cent union rate for acute unstable fractures (which they grafted if there was flexion collapse), and 83 per cent overall, including non-unions.

These results are far superior to those of Maudsley and Chen,[40] Gasser[37] and the Mayo group,[28] all of whom used a cancellous lag screw. We would recommend the Herbert screw as the implant of choice for scaphoid fractures and their sequelae.

Intercarpal fusions

Faithful and Herbert[26] have performed 13 intercarpal fusions with the Herbert screw. Ten were scapholunate fusions for carpal instability. The fusion rate was 70 per cent in these cases. Graft was used, and cast immobilization was recommended postoperatively. The remaining intercarpal fusions united.

The elbow

Intra-articular fractures of the elbow region are fertile ground for the Herbert screw.

Radial head fractures

The first recorded radial head fracture was noted during the post mortem of a man who had jumped from the second storey of a house in 1834, killing himself and sustaining a fracture dislocation of the elbow. In 1905, with the advent of Roentgen's Rays, Thomas could write, 'Instead of it being an extremely rare fracture . . . it is a common one. There are more cases of this fracture, in the hands of a few skiagraphers in Philadelphia than the writers could find after a thorough search of the literature.'[41]

If confusion and controversy surround the scaphoid fracture, those of the radial head are, if anything, more controversial. There is no disagreement over the majority of radial head fractures, the undisplaced (Mason type I:[42] see Figure 8.10), which are managed by aspiration of the haematoma and early movement. The disputes are over the rarer displaced segmental (Type II) and comminuted (Type III) fractures. If McLaughlin's criteria[40] for surgery of the displaced segmental fractures are accepted, it may be time to extend Mason's classification, creating IIa and IIb groups. Hence, if there is less than 3 mm displacement or 30 degrees of angulation, treatment should be non-operative, by early mobilization, but if greater, surgery should be considered.

Heim and Trub,[43] in 1978, were the first to advocate internal fixation of radial head fractures using AO screws. According to Radin and Riseborough's criteria,[44] 82 per cent of Heim and Trub's patients had good (less than 10 degrees' loss of joint movement in any direction and no symptoms) or fair (up to 30 degrees' loss of motion with minor symptoms) results.

We feel that the Mason IIb segmental displaced fracture is the best indication for Herbert screw fixation (Figure 8.11). We have reviewed our first 25 patients with radial head fractures fixed with the Herbert screw (Table 8.1). Nine patients had Type IIb fractures and all had good results.

Intra-articular fractures are, however, often worse than they appear on radiographs, and this is certainly true of comminuted radial head fractures. Many have extensive fissuring of the articular cartilage and plastic deformation of the osteochondral shell. Only eight out of ten in our series had good results. Temporary Kirschner wires were needed to hold the fragments during reconstruction and there was often evidence of capitellar damage and even fragments of capitellum

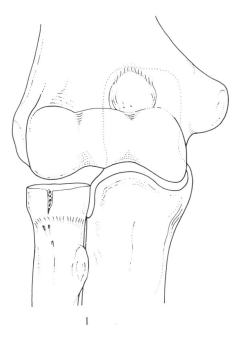

I

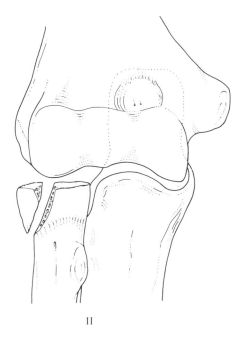

II

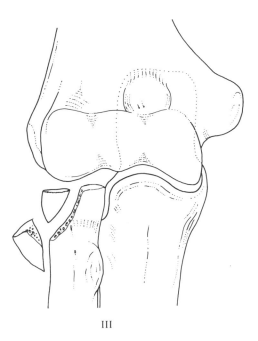

III

Figure 8.10 Mason's classification of radial head fractures.

jammed between the radial head fragments (Figure 8.12). Our results, although better than any other series of internal fixation of comminuted fractures, are not as good as those from excision of the radial head: if there is severe comminution fixation should not be considered, even with the aid of the Herbert differential pitch bone screw.

The course to be taken is, as yet, unresolved. Charnley,[45] advises against radial head excision. Adler and Shaftan[46] also championed non-operative treatment. They showed that this treatment was as good as, if not better than, excision, although there were too few patients in either group for statistical significance. Unfortunately, this was a retrospective study, the worst fractures having been treated operatively and the fracture dislocations (which have a much worse prognosis) added to the results.

In comparison, Radin and Riseborough state, 'The results for fractures involving more than two-thirds of the radial head are so clear cut that we do not hesitate to recommend early total excision for this group'. Unfortunately, the table of their results does not show treatment of any fracture greater than two-thirds of the radial head conservatively. It is thus not clear how they came to their conclusions. Indeed, their results for excision and conservative treatment are the same.

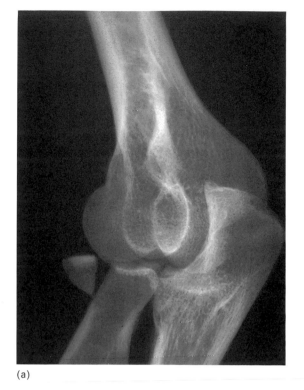

(a)

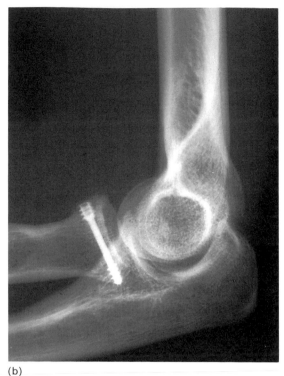

(b)

Figure 8.11 A segmental radial head fracture, *a*, before and, *b*, after fixation with the Herbert screw.

For their comminuted fractures, 20 out of 26 had less than good results following radial head excision.

Radial head fractures associated with postero-lateral dislocation of the elbow are often severely comminuted. Attempts at Nottingham to reassemble the radial head in six elbows, in order to restore some bone stability to the lateral side of the joint had poor results; notwithstanding, the injury itself has a poor prognosis in terms of joint stiffness. Ectopic bone formation is commonly associated with the extensive muscle damage, mainly to brachialis, occurring with this injury.

Table 8.1 Results of internal fixation of radial head fractures

Type	Number	Flexion	Pron/supination	% good
Undisplaced	0	—	—	—
Marginal displaced (Mason II)	9	6–136($\pm$5)	85($\pm$11)/84($\pm$8)	100
Comminuted (Mason III)	10	12–131($\pm$12)	88($\pm$6)/83($\pm$11)	80
Fracture dislocation (Mason IV)	6	30–125($\pm$19)	66($\pm$30)/75($\pm$28)	60

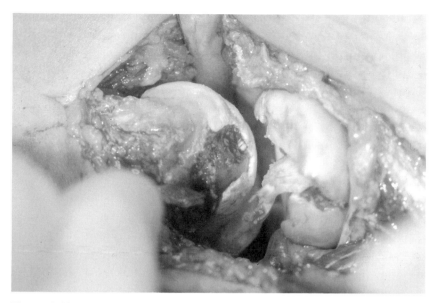

Figure 8.12 Fragments of capitellum tucked into a radial head fracture.

Capitellar fractures

Osteochondral fractures of the capitellum are much rarer than radial head fractures but are ideal cases for internal fixation with the Herbert screw (Figure 8.13). Although these fractures can be fixed, if the fragment is large enough, using a lag screw inserted from the posterior, non-articular surface of the capitellum, it is easier to use a Herbert screw inserted directly through the cartilage and buried beneath it. We have operated on five such cases. The radial head tends to lie directly on the reduced capitellum where the screw needs to be placed. For this reason, the screw has to be placed obliquely, using the freehand device. The results are good both radiologically and functionally, although some 20 degrees' loss of extension has been the norm.

Complex distal humeral fractures

The Herbert screw can be used to reconstruct small articular fragments in these extraordinarily difficult fractures. Figure 8.14 shows the radiographs of a van driver who sustained, along with multiple other injuries, an open distal humeral fracture. The articular surface was reconstructed well and post-operative function was flexion of 35 degrees to 110 degrees at one year.

Femoral head fractures

Fractures of the femoral head are uncommon, usually resulting from high velocity trauma and often associated with other injuries to the hip joint.[47,48] Three patients sustained this severe injury. In one, there was an ipsi-lateral fracture of the femoral neck while a second suffered a posterior dislocation of the same hip with partial sciatic nerve palsy. All three fractures required open reduction and fixation with multiple Herbert screws (Figure 8.15).

In all three cases, the osteochondral fractures united, with good return of mobility at the hip (flexion to greater than 100 degrees). However, the patient with the femoral neck fracture showed signs of avascular necrosis one year after his accident.

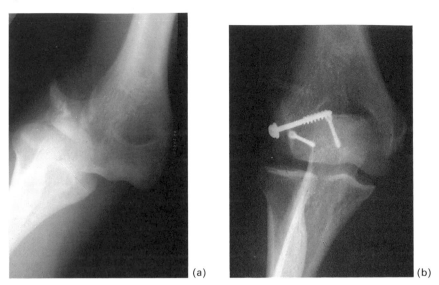

Figure 8.13 Capitellar fracture, *a*, before and, *b*, after fixation with the Herbert screw.

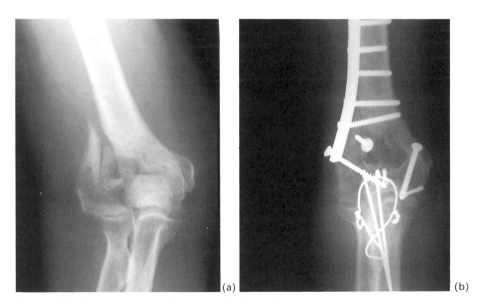

Figure 8.14 A complex humeral fracture, *a*, before and, *b*, after operative reconstruction.

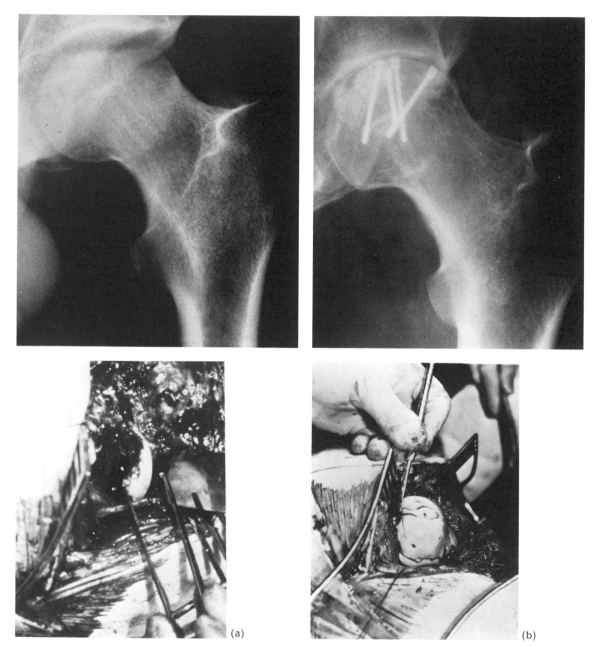

Figure 8.15 An osteochondral fracture of the femoral head, *a*, before and, *b*, after operation.

Osteochondral fractures of the knee

Of the six cases, five involved the lateral condyle and one the medial femoral condyle. The patients were followed up for an average of 12.3 months. At operation, all cases were found to have more articular cartilage damage than was expected from the pre-operative radiological examination. Five of the cases were reduced after arthrotomy and held with one or more screws. One case of osteochondritis dissecans, which had not separated, was screwed in situ arthroscopically. Bony union was seen radiographically to have occurred in all cases (Figure 8.16). The range of knee flexion was 129 degrees ± 10 degrees SD at follow-up.

Fractures of the talus

Three cases were treated, two involving the dome and one the neck. The average follow-up was seven months. In both dome osteochondral fractures (Figure 8.17), a good result was achieved, one having full subtalar movement, and the other 75 per cent compared to the other side. The talar neck fracture was associated with an open tibial fracture which was internally fixed, but protected with plaster for six weeks. There was minimal subtalar movement at four and a half months.

Figure 8.16 An osteochondral fracture of the knee which had been screwed arthroscopically.

Figure 8.17 Two fractures of the talus, which achieved good subtalar movement postoperatively.

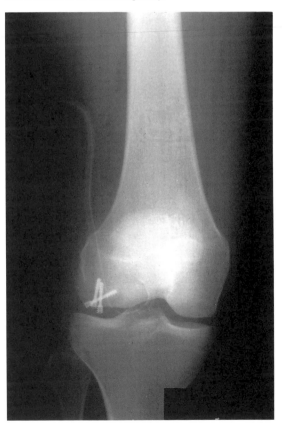

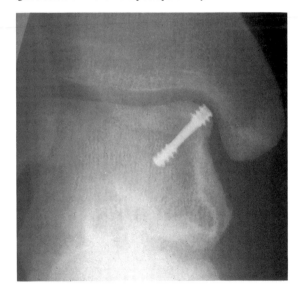

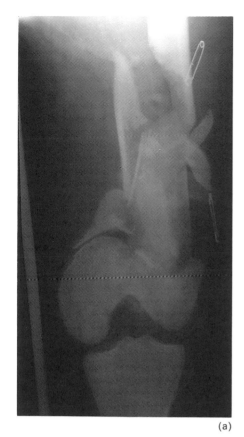

(a)

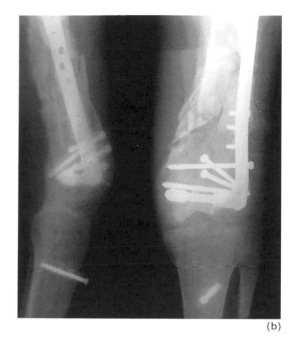

(b)

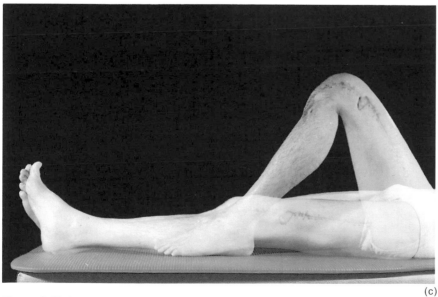

(c)

Figure 8.18 A supracondylar fracture of the knee, *a*, before and, *b*, after AO fixation involving Herbert screws, *c*, shows the result at six weeks.

Complex fixation

In three cases, Herbert screws were used as an adjunct to AO fixation (Figure 8.18). Two were supracondylar fractures of the femur, the third a comminuted fracture of the shaft of the tibia, where a small butterfly fragment was fixed in position using a Herbert screw. Bimetallic corrosion is a theoretical complication of complex fixation, between the titanium Herbert screws and the stainless steel AO screws.

Our current knowledge of cartilage healing, as discussed in this chapter, strongly suggests that optimal results will be achieved with accurate reduction of the osteochondral fracture with inter-fragmentary compression. The Herbert bone screw now makes this possible. The differential pitch allows for interfragmentary compression, the trailing thread can be totally buried beneath the articular surface, and its small size allows more than one screw to be used, even in areas as small as the radial head or scaphoid. Rigid fixation can be followed by early joint movement to improve cartilage nutrition and repair.

9

Management of proximal humeral fractures

W. A. Wallace, MB, BS, FRCS Ed,
FRCS Ed Orth
T. D. Bunker, BSc, MB, BS, MCh Orth,
FRCS, FRCS Ed

Undisplaced proximal humeral fractures are managed well with proper closed treatment, whereas severely displaced fractures are frequently troublesome to surgeon and patient alike. There is controversy both over whether to operate and over the kind and timing of operation. In order to try to answer some of these questions, certain facts must be considered.

Incidence and aetiology

Proximal humeral fractures are common (Table 9.1), about half as common as hip fractures, and account for 4 to 5 per cent of all fractures. It has been shown quite clearly by Horak and Nilsson[1] that the incidence rapidly increases with age, and that women are affected twice as often as men. The majority of series show a mean age of fracture at 67 years. The incidence in our group of 137 fractures[2] is shown in Figure 9.1; in

the distribution curve, the highest incidence occurs between 70 and 85 years of age. The only series with a low average age was that of Neer:[3] 117 patients, with three- and four-part fractures, had an average age of 55.3 years. Most patients sustaining proximal humeral fractures are over 80 years of age, with porotic bones indicative of 'insufficiency fractures', limited prospects and low rehabilitation drive. These factors should bias the surgeon against surgery in most, but not all, cases.

Classification

Neer's classic paper on the anatomical classification of proximal humeral fractures, in 1970,[4] should be read by all those interested in surgery of the shoulder. Neer based his classification on Codman's original description[5] of the four shoulder segments, and fortunately this classification has become almost universal.

Table 9.1 The incidence of proximal humeral fractures

Fracture type	Incidence/10,000 population/year	
Colles fracture	22	(Nottingham, 1986)
Hip fracture	8	(Nottingham, 1984)
Humeral neck fracture	3	(Tameside General Hospital, 1984)

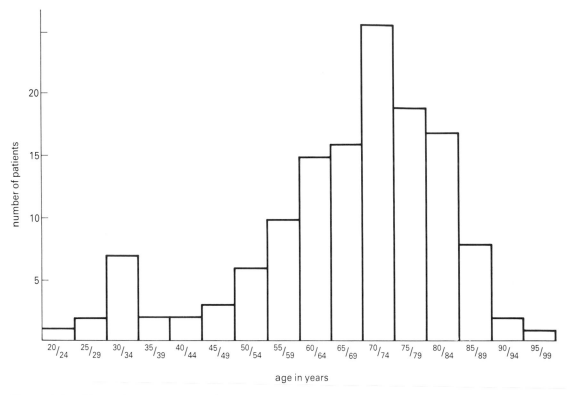

Figure 9.1 Incidence of proximal humeral fractures.

Objections have been raised that distinction between three- and four-part fractures can be difficult (Lundberg),[6] and that the grouping does not reflect the severity of prognosis, as group II fractures have a worse outcome than group III fractures (Jakob). Jakob and colleagues[7] have tried to overcome this latter difficulty by introducing an AO classification based on the AO grouping of fracture severity (A, B and C), with group A having the best outcome and group C, the intracapsular fractures, the worst. It is, however, unlikely that surgeons who have recently become used to one complex classification (Neer's) will be prepared to change to another, even more complex one.

Neer's classification (Figure 9.2)[8] is based on the following guidelines:

1. All undisplaced fractures fall into group 1.

2. The four-part classification refers only to fractures that have *parted* (displaced) by over 1 cm, or angulated by over 45 degrees.

In our study of 150 patients, 42 per cent had undisplaced fractures and 48 per cent had two-part fractures. This left only 10 per cent of truly severe three- and four-part fractures. Since nine out of every ten proximal humeral fractures are undisplaced or two-part fractures, it is vital that they are managed correctly.

Undisplaced fractures

Nearly all undisplaced fractures (94 per cent) have a very good outcome if the following four rules are observed:

1. Exclude associated dislocation with a good axial or lateral radiograph

2. Relieve pain by analgesia and support

3. Mobilize early

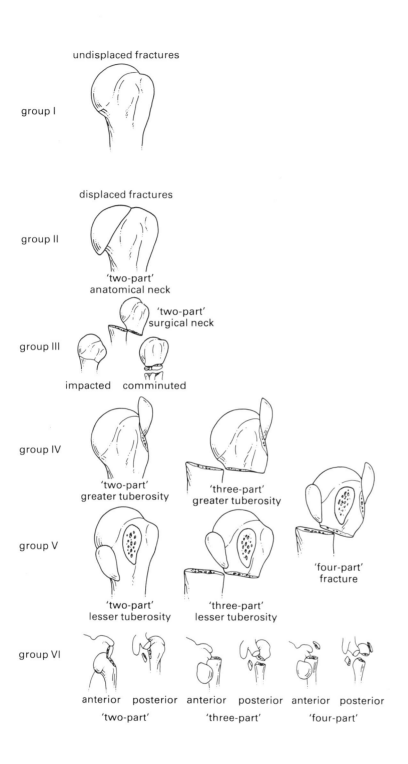

undisplaced fractures

group I

displaced fractures

group II

'two-part'
anatomical neck

'two-part'
surgical neck

group III

impacted   comminuted

group IV

'two-part'
greater tuberosity

'three-part'
greater tuberosity

group V

'four-part'
fracture

'two-part'
lesser tuberosity

'three-part'
lesser tuberosity

group VI

anterior   posterior   anterior   posterior   anterior   posterior

'two-part'   'three-part'   'four-part'

Figure 9.2 Neer's classification of undisplaced and
displaced fractures of two-, three- and four-part types.

4. Recognize that patients over 80 years of age rarely complain of stiffness but report pain as the major long-term problem.

All trauma surgeons recall cases of missed posterior dislocation of the shoulder, where a physician had interpreted the radiograph as a fracture of the proximal humerus. This can be disastrous for the patient. If a true axial radiograph cannot be obtained, either a lateral radiograph of the scapular plane, as described by Neer,[8] or a modified axial view,[9] can easily be obtained without the arm being removed from the sling. The modified axial view (Figure 9.3) gives a distorted view of the upper humeral shaft, but clearly demonstrates the relationship between humeral head and glenoid (Figure 9.4).

Pain may be caused by downward subluxation secondary to muscular inhibition of the rotator cuff and deltoid, and reduction of the subluxation using a supportive triangular sling for the first week (followed by a collar and cuff sling) will control it. Pain during the night is very distressing, and patients often insist that, for the first few days, it is better to sleep sitting in an armchair than lying in bed, which tends to angulate the fracture posteriorly.

Clifford[10] showed that the longer a sling was worn the poorer was the result, as early movement is most important. Outpatient physiotherapy is not required for most patients. Lundberg[11] has clearly demonstrated that patients taught to exercise at home show just as good results as those under regular outpatient physiotherapy. Most physiotherapy departments have developed their own exercise plans to help patients. Figure 9.5 illustrates the shoulder movement exercises started from day two and Figure 9.6 the muscle strengthening exercises, begun three weeks after hospitalization, used at the Nottingham Hospitals.

Displaced anatomical neck fractures

These fractures are extremely rare. Neer[8] admits that he does not have enough experience of them to be

Figure 9.3 Position of the patient and X-ray equipment in obtaining the modified axial view of the shoulder.

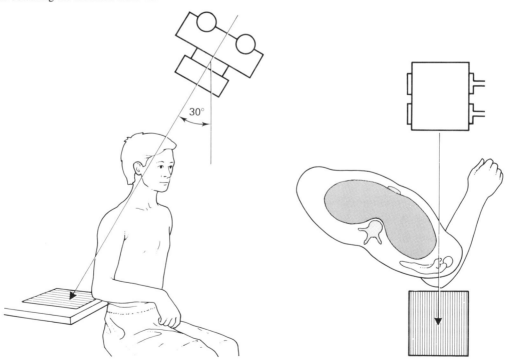

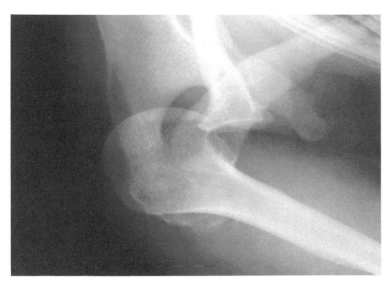

Figure 9.4 Distortion of humerus on a modified axial view.

dogmatic about their treatment. He states that malunion may be greater than originally anticipated from the initial radiographs, and that the fracture is associated with a high incidence of avascular necrosis. Blood supply of the humeral head derives mainly from the ascending branch of the anterior circumflex humeral artery, which rises up the lesser tuberosity in the bicipital sulcus. In this fracture, the humeral head must be devascularized, and it has been suggested that the vascular supply is replaced by creeping substitution as in the femoral head. Drawing the analogy with displaced subcapital fractures further, the best results are associated with the most accurate reduction (allowing a surface as large as possible for creeping substitution) and internal fixation. Should the same method be used on the humerus? Neer certainly thinks so, and advises open reduction and internal fixation.

Two-part displaced surgical neck fractures

There is controversy as to whether fracture fixation should be carried out, and if so, of what kind. Comparison of results is hampered by the small number of reviews of severe proximal humeral fractures and the different methods of assessing them.

One of the many advances in shoulder surgery introduced by Neer, is the 'Neer score'.[4] This has been adopted by many surgeons for the assessment of fractures around the shoulder (Figure 9.7). A score of less than 70 is considered poor, 70 to 79 is unsatisfactory, 80 to 90 is satisfactory, and a score of over 89 is considered excellent. However, some surgeons believe that this scoring system is too harsh, as in the worst fractures even the best results are graded as poor. Young and Wallace[12] state that the functional requirements in the elderly are only 60 degrees' abduction and an ability to raise the arm above the head and to the mouth; such results on their own would give a poor Neer score. Tanner and Cofield[13] and Stableforth[14] stress the need for adequate internal rotation for perineal hygiene; on the Neer score, internal rotation is given only two points, and perineal hygiene is not mentioned. Since elimination of pain is the main object of management of proximal humeral fractures, some surgeons feel that 35 out of 100 is not enough and that pain control should be scored separately. There is obviously an urgent need for agreement among shoulder surgeons about shoulder assessment after fracture.

What are the indications for surgery? Angulation on its own is not sufficient in two-part fractures. De Palma and Cantilli[15] showed that malunion became less pronounced during healing, and this has been confirmed by Young and Wallace.[12] The usual neck shaft angle is 140 degrees, and Paavolainen[16] has

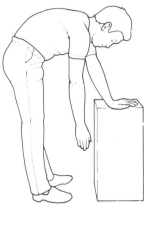

Figure 9.5 Shoulder movement exercises.

(i) Stand beside a firm support, for example, table or kitchen sink, lean with hand of *unaffected* arm on table, stoop forward as far as possible, let your arm hang *loosely* away from body, then swing arm in three directions: a. Moving backwards and forwards, as far as possible. b. Out to the side and back across the body, as far as possible. c. Circular movement.

(ii) Either sit or stand, clasp both hands together, straighten both elbows and raise arm above the head or as high as possible so that unaffected arm helps the affected one. Lower slowly. Relax.

(iii) Stand *facing* a wall or door with a slippery surface, place a duster under the hand of the affected arm, slide hand up the wall as far as possible, using the other arm to assist if necessary. Lower slowly. Relax.

(iv) Stand *sideways* to a wall or door, with a duster under the hand of the affected arm, slide arm upwards as high as possible. Lower slowly. Relax.

Check that your elbow *bends and straightens fully*, also that wrist and hand move fully. You should be able to perform most light chores, such as washing-up, and window cleaning.

Lifting of heavy objects should not be attempted initially; it is best to increase the weight lifted gradually.

Remember, when dressing it is much easier to insert the affected arm into sleeves first.

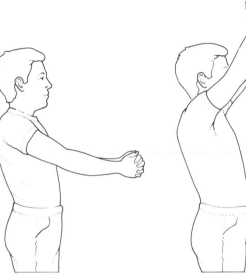

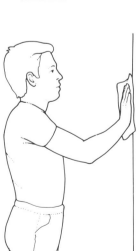

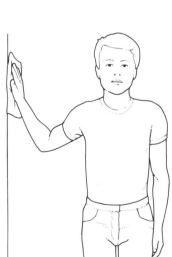

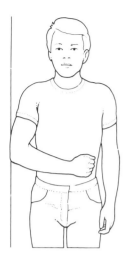 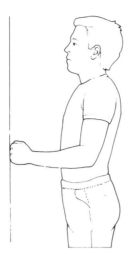 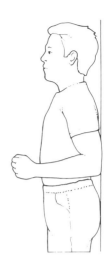

Figure 9.6 Shoulder strengthening exercises.
(i) Stand *sideways* to a wall, bend the elbow, place the elbow against the wall slightly away from the body. Press the elbow outwards against the wall *as hard as you can*. Relax. Take care *not* to use body weight, push only with elbow; you should feel tension in the shoulder muscle.
(ii) *Face* the wall, bend the elbow, make a fist, press the fist to the wall as hard as possible. Relax. Again, check that body weight is *not* used.
(iii) Stand with your *back* to the wall, bend the elbow, place the back of the elbow to the wall and press as hard as possible. Relax.

Check that your elbow bends and straightens fully, also that the wrist and hand move fully. These can all become stiff if your arm is not being used normally. You should be able to perform most light chores, such as washing-up and window cleaning. Lifting of heavy objects should not be attempted initially; it is best to increase the weight lifted gradually.

Remember, when dressing it is much easier to insert the affected arm into sleeves first. The exercises will be most effective if practised regularly, for example, repeating a few times every hour is much better than one long session daily.

shown that over 40 degrees of varus gives sub-acromial impingement with a bad outcome. The major indication for surgery is minimal or no bone contact associated with a high incidence of non-union. All five patients in the Young and Wallace series[12] who had the fracture manipulated for a 'no contact' fracture, without any form of fixation, had further displacements. This common finding means that bone apposition must be held until fracture union occurs. Fractures are held mostly with Rush pins, percutaneous Kirshner wires, AO 'T' plating or the Mouradian modified Zickel apparatus. The first two of these techniques will be described here, and the latter two will be discussed in the context of complex three- and four-part fractures, for which they are especially suited.

Rush pins

Historically, Rush pins, inserted closed through the tuberosities and across the fracture, have been very popular. However, there are few large series describing the results of this technique. Weseley, Barenfield and Eisenstein[17] performed Rush pinning on 16 patients within a period of 14 years. During that time they treated non-operatively over 700 patients with proximal humeral fractures. The semiclosed procedure, as described by Rush,[18] was used: one finger was inserted through a short deltopectoral incision to reduce the fracture. These authors cite several advantages for Rush pinning, particularly its ease, speed and limited morbidity. There were no non-unions or implant failures, and early mobilization prevailed.

The major criticism of this method is the inevitable damage of the superior part of the rotator cuff. This is the part of the cuff with the poorest blood supply and at most risk of rupture, but despite this the results were very good. The Rush pin should be removed at

FUNCTIONAL ASSESSMENT KEY							

1. PAIN — TOTAL 35

a)	NO PAIN	35
b)	Slight or occasional	30
c)	Mild, no effect in ordinary activity	25
d)	Moderate, tolerable, starting to affect ordinary activity	15
e)	Marked serious limitations of ordinary activity	5
f)	Total disablement	0

2. FUNCTIONAL ABILITY: — TOTAL 30

a) Strength		b) Reaching		c) Stability	
Normal	10	Above head	2	Lifting	2
Good	8	Mouth	2	Throwing	2
Fair	6	Belt buckle	2	Carrying	2
Poor	4	Opposite axilla	2	Pushing	2
Trace	2	Brassiere hook	2	Hold overhead	2
Zero	0				

3. RANGE OF MOTION — TOTAL 25

Flexion		Extension		Abduction		External Rotation (elbow bent)	
180	6	45	3	180	6	60	5 bent
170	5	30	2	170	5	30	3
130	4	15	1	140	4	10	1
100	2			100	2		
80	1			80	1		
<80	0	<15	0	<80	0	<10	0

INTERNAL ROTATION (elbow bent)		ANATOMY — TOTAL 10	
90 (T6)	5	Rotation, angulation, joint incongruity, retracted tuberosities, non-union, avascular necrosis.	
70 (T12)	4	None	10
50 (L5)	3	Mild	8
30 (glutea)	2	Moderate	4
>30	0	Severe	0–2
		TOTAL SCORE	100 RESULT
		>89	Excellent
		80	Satisfactory
		70	Unsatisfactory
		<70	Poor

Figure 9.7 Neer's classification of function following shoulder injury.

an early stage, once progress of fracture union becomes apparent on radiography. Unfortunately, removal of the pin is often more difficult than insertion, and in the elderly patient it is often left in situ (Figure 9.8).

Percutaneous Kirschner wires

Temporary K wires have been used by Jakob, Lundberg[6] and ourselves. Jakob states that, 'Although this technique may appear deceptively simple ... it is indeed very demanding and should only be used by an experienced surgical team as a useful alternative to open reduction and internal fixation.'[7]

The patient is positioned laterally, with the affected shoulder uppermost. A 'C arm' image intensifier (or preferably two intensifiers) are used to obtain biplanar imaging of the shoulder. In these fractures, the deforming force is the muscle pull of pectoralis major, overcome by traction applied by an experienced assistant (Figure 9.9).

Three stout K wires are then placed upwards from

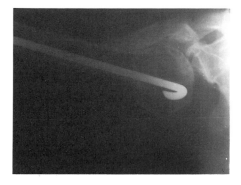

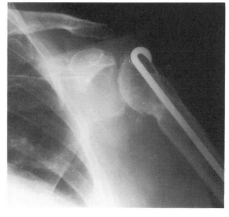

Figure 9.8 Rush pins inserted to hold two-part fracture.

the upper humeral shaft into the humeral head. Damage to either the axillary or radial nerves caused by the K wire is a recognized risk and a knowledge of the detailed anatomy and surface marking of these nerves is essential. For this reason, the best entry site is anteriorly, above the deltoid insertion. One problem is that the wires tend to skid off the humeral shaft, making insertion difficult. Damage to the rotator cuff is avoided by distal-to-proximal pin insertion, although occasionally a pin has to be passed in the opposite direction. Proximal pins should be removed at three weeks and distal pins at six weeks. The reduced fracture position was maintained in all patients in Lundberg's series, with pin track infection in two cases, which healed after removal of the wires. In Jakob's series,[7] 35 of 40 cases proceeded to union uneventfully, with only minimal deformity; many of those were more severe than two-part fracture cases (Figure 9.10).

Sometimes, closed reduction is not possible owing to interposition of the long head of biceps tendon, rendering open reduction necessary.

Two-part displaced greater tuberosity fractures

These fractures constitute 10 per cent of proximal humeral fractures.[2] This injury is the bony reflection

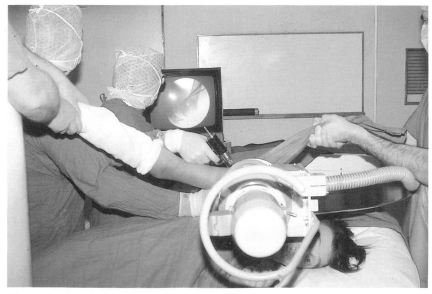

Figure 9.9 Traction during the insertion of the wires.

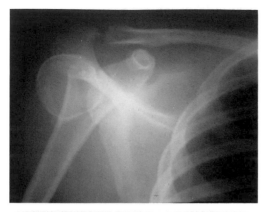

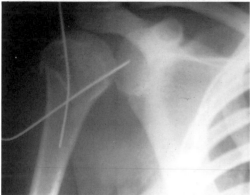

Figure 9.10 Fracture dislocation reduced and held with the wires.

of a torn rotator cuff, and if the greater tuberosity is left displaced it will cause blocking of elevation and abduction. For the majority of cases, the treatment of choice is open reduction through a small deltoid splitting or transacromial incision followed by stabilization with cancellous lag screws or interosseous suture. Even appropriate fixation with a 6.5 mm AO cancellous screw may give impingement from the screw head on the coracoacromial arch (Figure 9.11).

Thus, interosseous suturing, although old-fashioned, has its place in this particular situation, which should be regarded as a rotator cuff disruption rather than a fracture. Drill holes of 3.5 mm are made in both fragments, and Number 2 Ethibond is used to effect a repair that is strong and smooth enough not to cause subacromial impingement. Wire is no longer recommended, as fragmentation may later cause damage to the joint (Figure 9.12).

The timing of surgery is important: within four days from the time of fracture, or after four weeks when soft tissues are less bruised and swollen and more amenable to careful repair.

In some patients, for cosmetic reasons, it is justifiable to treat this injury with an 'aeroplane' splint in abduction, but only if the reduction in the splint is absolutely correct anatomically and remains so through the six week period to union.

Three- and four-part fractures, or fracture dislocations

These uncommon fractures occur in only 11 per cent of cases,[2] but their management is highly controversial. Before the results of surgical intervention are considered, their natural history as a baseline needs to be discussed. Neer[3] found only three satisfactory results in 77 patients managed by closed reduction, and Clifford reported poor results in nine out of 19 cases at two years.[10] One explanation for these poor results is that they were scored on the extremely critical Neer system. We have found that, on a careful radiological review, conservatively treated three-part fractures improve their anatomical alignment. The majority of these fractures occur in elderly women in whom the acceptable objectives are 60 degrees' abduction, ability to raise the arm above the head, behind the neck and behind the back, satisfaction with the usefulness and power of the limb and, most importantly, elimination of pain. (All three of our patients with three-part fractures had acceptable results.) Of Leyshon's 34 patients with three-part fractures, 24 had satisfactory results using Neer's scoring system, and this would agree with our findings. However, all four-part fractures had poor results.[19] Stableforth[14] had extremely poor results from non-operative treatment of these fractures and fracture dislocations: of 32 patients, only one had no pain, only six could bring their hand to their mouth, while seven patients were totally dependent and nine were partially dependent on others for simple activities of daily living. In Stableforth's prospective study of surgery versus non-operative management, nine out of 12 patients were in constant pain and only seven out of 16 were leading an independent life six months following injury. It is against this background that operative intervention should be judged. Most authors would agree that operative intervention means fixation for three-part fractures, and hemiarthroplasty or fixation for four-part fractures.

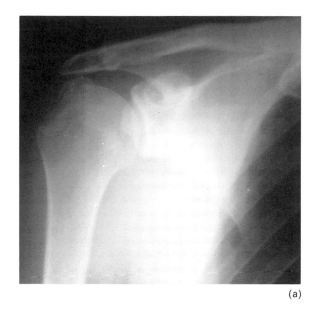

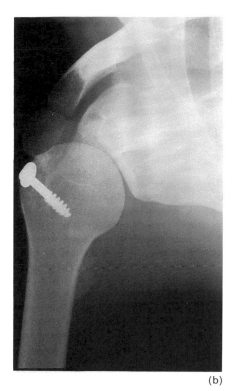

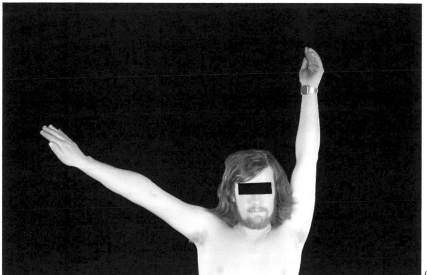

Figure 9.11 *a* Fracture of the greater tuberosity; *b* held with a single screw; *c* leading to subacromial impingement.

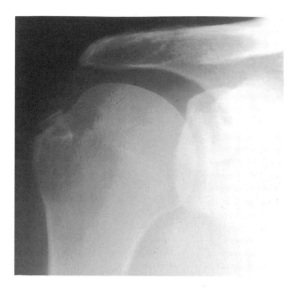

Figure 9.12 Greater tuberosity fracture reduced and sutured with interosseous sutures.

AO plating

The surgical method most commonly used is Neer's long deltopectoral approach.[20] The arm is abducted at 90 degrees and placed on an arm-table; this brings the deltopectoral line above the humeral head and consequently there is no need to divide any of the anterior fibres of the deltoid. Even more versatile is the modified extensile approach:[21] the anterior one-third of the clavicle bearing the anterior deltoid origin is osteotomized, leaving the posterior two-thirds of the clavicle intact. The deltoid is then hinged forward on the acromioclavicular joint, allowing a superb view of the proximal humerus. Osteotomy can be securely replaced at the end of the procedure, allowing rapid postoperative rehabilitation (Figure 9.13).

Paavolainen et al reported the results of operation on 41 patients using the AO technique.[16] On Neer's scoring system, 74 per cent had an excellent or satisfactory result. All patients of working age except one returned to work within four months. The most common technical error was positioning the AO plate too high, with a persistent varus deformation of the head. No patient developed avascular necrosis, but one had deep infection.

Kristiansen and Christensen[22] produced less satisfactory results from AO buttress plating. Although the technique offered satisfactory reduction, good stability and no non-unions, there was a high incidence of complications. These included two cases of deep infection, five plate impingements or loosening requiring plate removal, and four cases of avascular necrosis. They concluded that AO plating should be avoided in the elderly, and only undertaken by experienced surgeons.

Modified Zickel apparatus

In the originator's hands,[23] the Mouradian modified Zickel apparatus has given good results (average Neer score 83) in three- and four-part fractures. This may become the method of choice for three-part fractures, but the series was selected because patients over 60 years of age were treated by hemiarthroplasty and thus were excluded from the study.

Figure 9.13 A T plate for fixation of proximal humeral fracture.

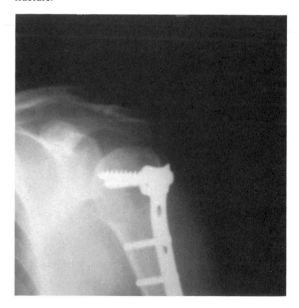

When carrying out internal fixation, it is important to remember that the bone stock is usually poor, and bone grafting with cancellous graft packed into the humeral head is recommended in all cases.

Postoperative management is important. The aim of surgery is to obtain stable fixation, to allow early movement, and physiotherapy ideally should begin at two days and be supervised for four weeks.

Fracture dislocation injuries

These rare but severe injuries are often associated with neurological or vascular damage. An attempt to reduce three- or four-part fracture dislocations should never be made under sedation alone, and general anaesthesia is mandatory. Reduction should be performed with skill and care, using direct pressure on the head fragment and never a rotational manoeuvre, as this may worsen the state of the fracture. Radiographs (anteroposterior and lateral) should then be taken with the patient anaesthetized and further treatment would be based on the per-operative appearance.

If closed reduction cannot be effected, the procedure should be abandoned and arrangements made for open management when ideal theatre facilities are available, including a full set of AO implants and Neer prostheses.

Figure 9.14 Mark I Neer hemiarthroplasty three months after four-part fracture dislocation.

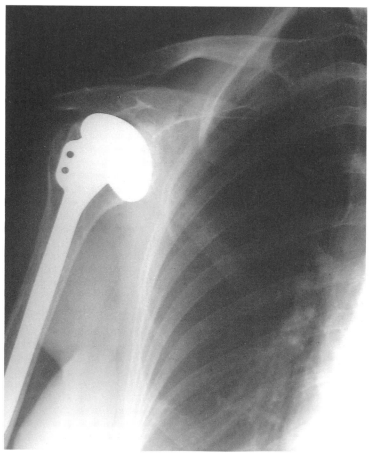

In Neer's series,[3] there were no satisfactory results for four-part fractures treated 'closed' or with open reduction, and there were nine cases of avascular necrosis in 24 patients. Leyshon showed no satisfactory results in four-part fractures.[19] Surgical reconstruction often fails owing to avascular necrosis, and excision of the head leads to poor function (Knight and Mayne).[24] It is against this background that hemiarthroplasty needs to be considered.

Neer obtained 'satisfactory but imperfect' results from hemiarthroplasty with an average score of 82.[3] However, his patients had an average age of 55 years.

Stableforth,[14] in a randomized study of conservative management versus hemiarthroplasty in four-part fractures, showed greater mobility in the hemiarthroplasty group, with 11 patients able to flex over 90 degrees compared with only one in the conservative group. He also noted more constant pain in the conservative group (nine patients) compared with the hemiarthroplasty group (two patients), and concluded that Neer replacement had significant advantages over conservative management (Figure 9.14).

However, in a number of centres there is dissatisfaction with hemiarthroplasty because of the associated poor results. Des Marchais and colleagues[25] reported that 11 of 29 patients had unsatisfactory results from hemiarthroplasty, nine of which were probably due to rotator cuff disruption. Kraulis and Hunter[26] achieved good results in only two of 13 patients, and the local and general complication rate was high (however, one-third of their patients were chronic alcoholics). Willems and Lim[27] reported unsatisfactory results following hemiarthroplasty in six out of ten cases, and noted very marked postoperative glenohumeral stiffness. Again, this emphasizes the strictness of the Neer score for all patients, except one, who showed no restriction in daily activities, with only one patient in pain. Hirst and Wallace[28] reported unsatisfactory results owing to rotator cuff disruption in three of six patients.

Of the Neer Mark II implants, only the 22 mm head prosthesis should be used for acute fracture work, as there is usually no significant rotator cuff deficiency; however, there is often metaphyseal comminution.

It cannot be stressed enough that, in surgery around the shoulder, the soft tissues are most important: great care should be taken not only to repair the rotator cuff, but also to correct humeral length so as to achieve correct tension in the rotator cuff and deltoid. To this end, if there is metaphyseal comminution, the prosthesis may need to be anchored with bone cement not only to ensure the correct 30 to 40 degrees of retroversion, but also to maintain humeral length.

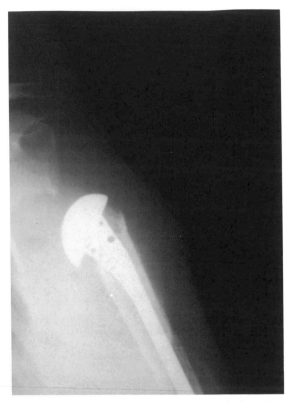

Figure 9.15 Too much emphasis on the prosthesis and not enough on the soft tissues leads to a poor result.

Too much emphasis was placed in the past on insertion of the artificial humeral head, with little importance attached to reconstruction of the rotator cuff. Figure 9.15 shows a typical poor result deriving from this misconception.

Conclusion

Surgical intervention for humeral neck fractures is difficult, and should not be carried out without good operating facilities and radiological support. There is strong evidence in published research for the use of humeral hemiarthroplasty in the elderly, particularly for four-part fractures and fracture dislocations. However, some surgeons have not been entirely satisfied with the final outcome, and have become more cautious with experience.

10

Functional bracing

D. I. Rowley, MB, ChB, B Med Biol, MD, FRCS

It is often said that nothing is new in medicine, and functional bracing is no exception to this. Although much of the history outlined below appears to bear this aphorism out, it is an illusion. Functional bracing is a new philosophy that can be traced to a handful of recent antecedents.

Early examples of splints attributed to Benjamin Googe of Norwich in 1777 bear an uncanny resemblance to modern femoral and tibial braces (Figure 10.1a). Gavil Wilson's leather patellar-bearing splint of 1801 could be said to have pre-empted Sarmiento by over a century (Figure 10.1b). However, these examples really serve to demonstrate the considerable difficulties encountered by early practitioners when it came to choosing casting materials.

Hippocrates and the Arabs used resins and egg white mixed with lime. Immobilization was often achieved by setting the limb in a block of material moulded in a box. This must have been both heavy and hazardous. It was not until the early nineteenth century that a Dutch army surgeon, Antoninus Mathysen, demonstrated that calcium sulphate hemihydrate combined with cotton bandage could be moulded when wet and then allowed to set to form a splint.

The facility of rigid immobilization using plaster of Paris contributed to a philosophy first formally put forward by John Hilton.[1] His principles, perpetuated by Hugh Owen Thomas,[2] dictated that rest of a fractured limb should be prolonged and enforced until union occurred. The concept that a broken limb, and the joint above and the joint below, should be so 'immobilized', has been a central dogma of orthopaedic surgery ever since.

In 1910 Championierre[3] wrote of the possibility of early active motion in the treatment of fractures, but he made little impression. The fundamental change in approach to conservative fracture treatment encompassed in cast bracing belongs to Augusto Sarmiento, who proposed his method for treating fractured tibiae in 1967.[4] Mooney et al[5] extended Sarmiento's ideas to apply to the femur with the introduction in 1970 of the metal-hinged femoral brace.

Since that time, developments can be largely attributed to advances in material technology. Thermoplastics allow braces to be made adjustable and so extend their use to a wider range of applications in fracture management. More novel materials including polyurethane and glass fibre laminates and polyvinyl acetate foams have resulted in lighter, cheaper and more manageable braces. Preformed cast braces are already available and the use of plastics and composites promises to improve this area of brace development.

How does a brace work?

Functional bracing permits the affected limb and the patient to function during the healing of a fracture. Braces are designed so that joints adjacent to the fracture are left free to move. It is fair to say that the practicalities of bracing preceded the realistic theory by some considerable time.

Sarmiento's original concept of a brace off-loading the fracture is probably too simple and immediately

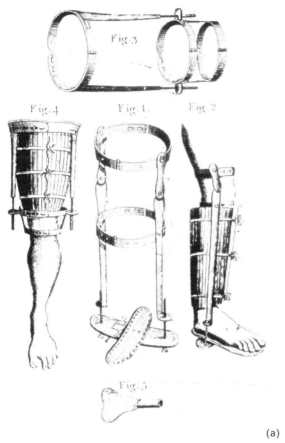

(a)

(b)

Figure 10.1 *a* Googe splints for the femur and the tibia;
b Wilson's leather patellar bearing splint.

fails to apply when braces other than that of the tibia
are considered. His own work on the tibial brace
complements the work of Meggitt and Thomas,[6] and
Wardlaw et al,[7] who analysed the role of the femoral
brace. They both concluded that although the brace
will support the fracture by approximately 30 per cent
of body weight, most of the off-loading of a lower
limb fracture is done by crutches during ambulation.
A fractured femur may be subjected to three times
body weight in normal walking, so the role of the
brace as a load-protecting device is minimal.

Sarmiento[8] has demonstrated that fractures encompassed in a brace do not shorten any more in the
splint than the degree of length loss noted at the time
of brace application, despite full weight bearing
(Figure 10.2). He proposes that the brace underpins
the tissues surrounding the fracture so the hydraulics

of the enclosed system support the fracture. Both
Sarmiento and Meggitt point out that the elastic
integrity of the soft tissues, particularly the fascia and
interosseous membrane, if present, will also contribute to fracture stability when the brace has been
applied.

There are certain objectives in the treatment of any
fracture in a containing splint:

1. Prevention of shortening and shift

2. Prevention of angulation of the distal fragment

3. Prevention of rotation at the fracture site.

This does not necessarily mean immobilization of the
limb. It is naïve to think that any splint, however well

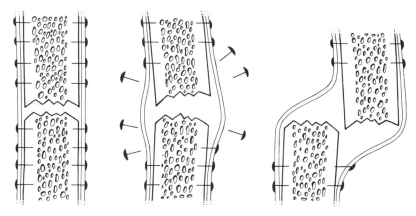

Figure 10.2 A simple analogy of shortening and the role of soft tissues may be drawn when considering a solid cylinder covered in paper held by tacks. As more tacks pull out, then the more unstable the rod becomes. However, the ultimate instability can be no worse than the number of tacks removed initially (after Sarmiento).

applied, will do more than control a fracture within certain limits.

The brace prevents shortening and shift in the way described above. Angulation is prevented by its rigid cylindrical nature. Rotation is prevented by careful moulding of the splint, so that it exactly fits the limb or even slightly compresses the soft tissues in certain areas. A brace may therefore be called a hydraulic antirotation device (Figure 10.3).

Rotatory control in the tibia is achieved by moulding the upper part of the brace around the calf, and some believe that rotatory control is enhanced by extension of the brace over the femoral condyles. Whether this is justified will be discussed below. In the

Figure 10.3 Rotatory control is achieved by triangulation in the upper tibia and by squaring off in the upper femur.

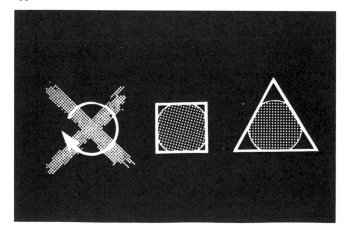

femur, the thigh portion of the brace is moulded into a snug-fitting quadrilateral shape at the top to control the rotation of the upper femoral fragment. Similar examples may be described for other functional braces used to treat other fractures. The important principle is that the brace must fit closely to the part it is designed to control all the time, or its function will be severely impaired.

This is a tall order and demands constant attention at follow-up if disasters are to be avoided. If limbs are braced too early, the oedema will result in a poor-fitting brace, as it disperses on mobilization. Too tight a fit on a wasted limb may prejudice the outcome when muscles begin to hypertrophy. The implication is clear—a brace must be fitted well initially and its design must allow for subsequent adjustment in situ by the patient or the therapist to guarantee an intimate fit at all times.

Indications

There are four situations where bracing is possible. The first is straightforward but the others are controversial:

1. Low velocity midshaft long bone fractures

2. High velocity midshaft fractures

3. Periarticular fractures (including the forearm)

4. In support of poor internal fixation.

Low velocity midshaft fractures

Tibial fractures

The tibia has enjoyed a general popularity among bracing enthusiasts since Sarmiento first described it in 1967.[4] From the development of the patellar-bearing plaster material, technology has now led to the production of preformed braces made of polythene and customized adjustable polyurethane braces (described below). Sarmiento[9] has recently reported the results of treating 625 diaphyseal tibial fractures over a period of five years. He describes less than a centimetre of shortening in over 90 per cent and an angular deformity of less than 5 degrees in 80 per cent. His series included a number of open injuries, and although he does not comment on the energy of injury, it would appear to be a series reflecting a complete spectrum of tibial injuries. He presents a non-union rate of 2.5 per cent, which is well within

average for tibial fractures. To anyone who has visited Professor Sarmiento's unit, these figures are remarkable because his group treats patients from some of the most socially deprived areas in the United States.

Such figures are impressive but they do involve a number of pitfalls for the unwary. If the fibula is intact, the fracture may tend to drift to varus and this may occur quite late, many weeks after bracing. This is not a contraindication to bracing; neither are fractures of the upper third of the tibia, unless the fibula is intact. In the latter situation, Sarmiento would avoid bracing, although in a Sheffield series of over fifty such fractures the problem was overcome by using a femoral, hinged brace. In the lower third tibial fracture, it may be preferable to delay bracing to avoid anterior tibial bowing. Such fractures may be treated in a classical patellar-bearing cast for a few weeks, to permit soft tissue consolidation before progressing to a brace with an ankle articulation (Figure 10.4).

Femoral bracing

Although Roper[10] used femoral hinged braces at the London Hospital earlier, widespread interest in the technique may be attributed to the work of Mooney et al in 1970.[5] Since then, femoral bracing has enjoyed a mixed popularity. There has always been a suspicion among practitioners that the femur will shorten and angulate. Connolly and King[11] appear to have demonstrated telescoping using radiographic techniques but there is little general support for their viewpoint elsewhere in the literature. Indeed, it is possible to argue that repeated pistoning of fracture fragments, as long as it is not excessive, may positively aid bony union.

Biomechanical analyses by Meggitt and Thomas[6] and by Wardlaw et al[7] have demonstrated that femoral fractures can be adequately controlled in braces. The lower third fracture is particularly suited to bracing as alternative operative treatments are less than satisfactory. The medullary canal in this region is too flared to hold a conventional nail and onlay plates are at significant risk from fracture. Alternative operative approaches are available but rely on high technology, such as radiological placement of cross bolts through bone and nail. Such techniques are excessively difficult and are unlikely to be universally adopted.

The midshaft femur is amenable to bracing and providing fracture position has been maintained on traction—by no means an easy feat—bracing is as good a method as surgical fixation. The upper third fracture is more contentious. Even using a pelvic band and maintaining an initial valgus position of the distal

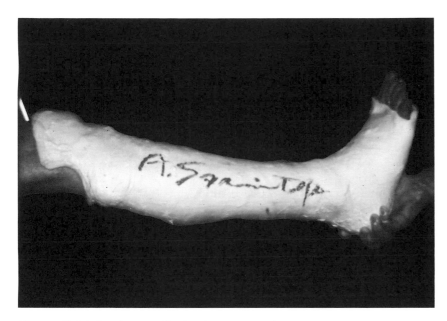

Figure 10.4 A Sarmiento patellar-bearing cast as made by Sarmiento during an impromptu teaching session in Sheffield. Note the great height he achieves on the patellar boss while maintaining contact with the femur. This is the area least well emulated by Sarmiento's followers.

fragment, varus drift and shortening are frequently found. It has been the author's experience that braces should be reserved for the otherwise inoperable upper third fracture.

Humeral fractures

Fracture surgeons have been treating humeral shaft fractures by functional bracing techniques for many years, often without realizing it. A posterior slab and a firm bandage add support to soft tissues, which in turn hold the fracture. Sarmiento[12] has described a more formal method using a plastic cylinder. He describes 119 humeral shaft fractures treated in this way with only one non-union. This series includes 39 per cent of gunshot injuries.

Despite the ability of the humerus to compensate for malunion through mobility, malrotation and angulation should not be tolerated. In particular, varus and internal rotation deformities will cause considerable inconvenience when the arm is in the resting position. The lower third humeral fracture is particularly prone to this and so injury in this region

is often better treated operatively. Similarly, if the fracture is too high around the tuberosities, a splint is likely to act as a fulcrum about which a fracture may angulate (Figure 10.5).

High velocity midshaft fractures

From these arguments it is logical to conclude that in high velocity injuries, where soft tissues are extensively damaged, bracing may not be appropriate. Such injuries are extremely difficult to treat by whatever methods chosen and the more interventional the technique, the greater the risk. Bracing has the merit of being simple and relatively devoid of risk. Because it is a non-invasive technique, providing follow up is diligent the method can be abandoned early if it is failing, and other methods instituted.

There has recently been an explosion of interest in external fixation techniques for the treatment of severe injuries, as outlined elsewhere in this book. Bracing makes a useful adjuvant to rigid fixators and may be used once soft tissue injuries have been

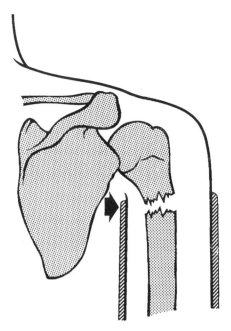

Figure 10.5 High fractures of the humerus should not be braced because of the tendency of the brace to distort the fracture.

controlled. The use of braces, where soft tissue disruption is extensive, is a matter of judgment and timing. Late bracing may not be of direct benefit to the fracture but it may still permit early mobilization of the patient and his joints.

Periarticular fractures

There can be no greater controversy than over the use of braces around joints where there is a close correlation between structure and function. According to modern teaching, in this relationship it is logical to restore anatomy precisely, to provide the best chance of perfect restoration of function. However logical this theory may seem, it has proved hard to confirm in practice.

There have been extensive recent advances in internal fixation and instrumentation has reached a high standard. There is no doubt that this progress has contributed significantly to improvements in fracture care, but the techniques are exacting, the risks great and the price of failure high. The rewards of successful internal fixation are early joint motion and a

restoration of movement with possibly a subsequent improved quality of cartilage repair of the joint.[13] It would be attractive to find a technique that maximizes the advantages of early joint motion but at less risk than internal fixation.

Functional bracing has been used to treat tibial plateau fractures and good results are reported by both Scotland and Wardlaw[14] and Beard et al.[15] There are limitations, and clearly gross joint destruction will preclude bracing. For example, lateral shear-type plateau fractures are better fixed, as late displacement is otherwise likely. However, comminuted compression type injuries are often almost impossible to fix and bracing here is an attractive alternative. Both groups mentioned above illustrate good or excellent results in over 90 per cent of fractures providing the depression of the plateau is less than 5–7 mm (Figure 10.6).

Internally fixed fractures

Theoretically it is wrong to immobilize fractures that have been fixed. The premises on which Mueller et al. justify internal fixation[16] include early mobilization without external splintage, so preventing 'fracture disease'. Functional bracing is based upon similar arguments, and so to combine the two would not appear to be logical. However, we do not live in a perfect world and it is often found that fixations, particularly in extreme situations and where bone quality is poor, are less than perfect. In these cases a functional brace may be used to augment internal fixation and so minimize the disadvantage of supporting insecure fixations with an exoskeleton.

Brace design

Casting materials

There is little doubt that recent advances in functional bracing are attributable as much to the availability of new and exciting materials as to changes in philosophy. Until recently, plaster of Paris was the only material available. This is brittle, heavy and rigid and permits no adjustment when set. A brace must be strong, light, slightly flexible and adjustable. Real advances were made with the production of thermoplastic sheets. These are now being slowly superseded by preformed plastic braces and braces made of polyurethane and glass fibre roll material.

Thermoplastic sheets consist either of isoprene rubbers and filler or polycaprolactones. Both materials

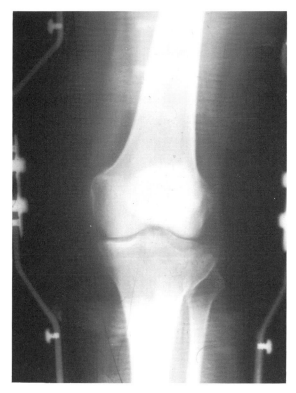

Figure 10.6 An anteroposterior radiograph of a lateral tibial plateau fracture treated in a femoral brace. The lateral radiograph has been omitted because the hinge obscures the view.

become soft at temperatures that may be tolerated next to the skin and set rapidly as they cool. They may be reheated and adjusted if the fit is not accurate and minor adjustments may be made in situ with a heat gun. They are not easy materials to use and the fitting of a brace is a time-consuming and labour intensive skill. This particular technique requires a number of pre-measurements and often practitioners make a paper cut-out first, rather like a tailor's template. Even in the best hands the method may take up to two hours.

Unfortunately the thermoplastics have not enhanced the acceptance of functional bracing. They are generally non-porous, despite having some perforations, so the skin is at risk from excoriation through sweating. For this reason the brace must be removable as well as adjustable. Early bracing may therefore not be possible. Besides, a great burden of trust is placed on patients with these braces, not to remove them. The materials' difficult handling characteristics when hot, particularly by tending to stick to themselves at the wrong moment, have not made them universally popular. Newer materials based on polyvinyl acetate foams overcome these problems by having an open cell configuration, but they remain largely untried in functional braces.

The polyurethane resins, usually in combination with glass fibre bandage, represent a true composite material that can be wound around the limb and allowed to set, forming a rigid laminate structure. These materials are strong, light, slightly flexible and can be made adjustable. They therefore fill all the design criteria of an ideal bracing material. They come as open mesh rolls and when formed into braces they are essentially porous and will freely permit passage of sweat while remaining intrinsically waterproof. Although flexible enough to permit a limited adjustment, they are too rigid for an opening to be made which would allow the braces to be removed without the danger of permanent deforming. However, as the materials are porous, skin excoriation is rarely a problem and by being adjustable but not removable braces made from them are less prone to patient abuse.

The physical properties of the bandage materials have been well investigated by a number of workers[17-19] and their superiority confirmed. They and the thermoplastics remain expensive but when compared to the costs of alternative treatments to bracing, they prove to be very economical.

Hinges

Braces for the femur, often for the tibia and occasionally fractures around the elbow, require a hinge. The knee presents particular difficulties for the engineer as it has a constantly varying axis of rotation (Figure 10.7a). The ankle too presents a problem because of the obliquity of its axis (Figure 10.7b), and only the elbow joint can realistically be treated as a simple hinge. A way around the difficulties has been to ignore the complexity of the joint axis and use a simple metal pivot, no more sophisticated than a door hinge. Such a solution will inevitably put strain on the relationship between brace and leg, which at best will weaken the hinge, or at worst damage the joint.

An alternative is the plastic hinge (Figure 10.8a), which essentially consists of a flexible bar of plastic or nylon that supports and aligns the cast brace components and otherwise bends mainly in flexion and extension in response to joint motion. Superficially

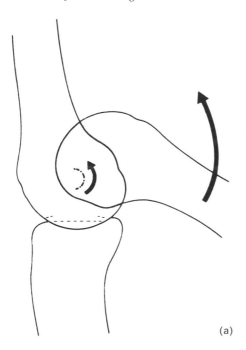

(a)

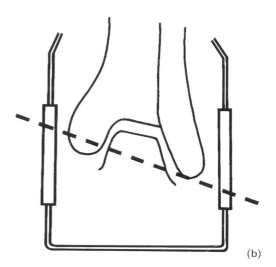

(b)

Figure 10.7 *a* Illustrates the variable instant centre pathway of rotation of the knee in the sagittal plane in a young and healthy individual; *b* illustrates the oblique axis of rotation of the ankle in the coronal plane. For simplicity, the axis may be said to lie along a line joining the two malleoli.

this may seem an acceptable compromise, but in reality it is a poor substitute. Plastic hinges require significant loads to make them bend and in early fracture management this may be undesirable. They are not good at preventing rotatory forces under load and they may permit the fracture to be subjected to high torques. They also tend to bow laterally under axial load and this may result in brace ridedown. If the brace is non-adjustable or the therapist fails to recognize the phenomenon, intimate contact between brace and limb is easily lost (Figure 10.8*b*).

A much better solution is to tackle the problem head-on by designing a hinge that will accommodate the variable instant centre pathway of the knee and the oblique axis of the ankle. If one hinge can do both and still act as a simple hinge about the elbow, so much the better. A programme of work conducted in Sheffield, Britain in conjunction with an industrial design company (Protectair Limited) followed such a line and a commercially available hinge system was produced that won a British Design Council award in 1986.

The Sheffield system works by providing a hinge with two axes of rotation (Figure 10.9*a*) that can also articulate about each other, rather like a three-link chain. Similar so-called 'polyaxial' hinges were previously available but their design is flawed because the two centres of rotation are linked together by cogs. This produces a virtually single-pivot hinge which does not follow the normal axis variation of the knee. The Sheffield hinge does not need a cog gearing to prevent collapse or 'zig-zag' of its mechanism because its front stop effectively controls the hinge's intrinsic alignment. The new hinge provides a window of available axis which will accommodate both the variable instant centre pathway of the knee and the oblique axis of the ankle without strain (Figure 10.9*b* and 9*c*).

Examples of braces

In the space available it would be impossible to give

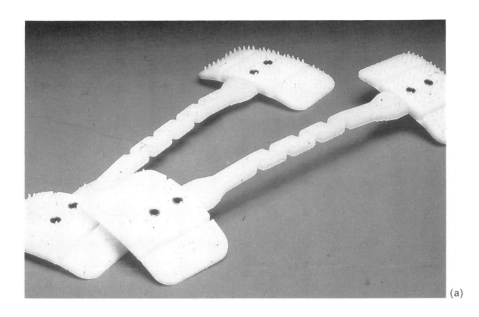

(a)

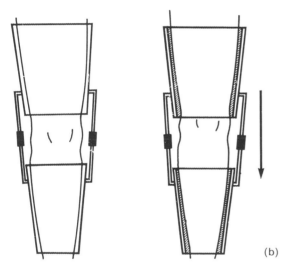

(b)

Figure 10.8 *a* Plastic bars often referred to as hinges: they flex and extend throughout their length in response to the joint motion. They are quite stiff enough to make movement awkward but not stiff enough to prevent brace ridedown *b*.

details of all types of braces using different materials. Therefore examples will be given of femoral, tibial, humeral and forearm braces using polyurethanes. The polyurethanes have been chosen because they represent future trends. They also offer the possibility

of a simple system which can be learned quickly and applied in any part of the world, whatever the climate. This is not to decry other materials with which readers are familiar. The principles illustrated by these examples are the same whatever the material used, with the exception of plaster of Paris. The author feels that plaster of Paris is inappropriate for a brace since it cannot be rendered adjustable.

The femoral brace (Figure 10.10)

The function of the upper component is to provide the hydraulic environment that will support the fracture. The upper third of the brace is shaped either by hand or with moulds to form a rounded quadrilateral, thereby ensuring rotatory control of the upper fracture fragment—a sort of reversed square peg in a round hole.

The lower component of the brace consists of the knee hinges and the calf piece. The ankle may be a continuation of the calf piece so that it is effectively a below-knee cast. The addition of an ankle hinge has the advantages of reducing jarring at heel strike and making walking less energy-consumptive. The function of the lower component is to support the brace—

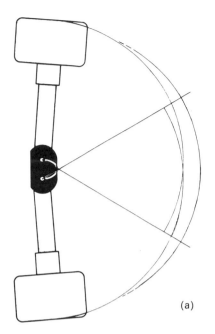

(a)

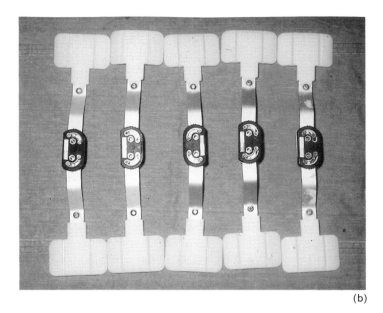

(b)

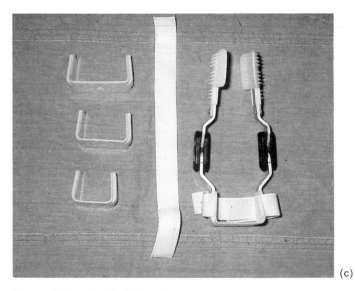

(c)

Figure 10.9 *a* The Sheffield bipivotal system permits an axis of motion anywhere in a window demarcated by a line drawn between the two pivots and a triangle subtended posteriorly as illustrated. *b* The hinges come in a range of prebent sizes for immediate fitting. *c* The same mechanism may be used in the ankle where the window of axis will encompass the obliquity of that of the ankle (compare with Figure 10.7).

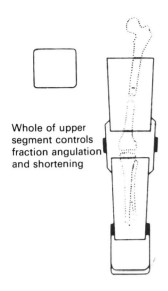

Quadrilateral shape
to control upper
fragment rotation

Whole of upper
segment controls
fraction angulation
and shortening

Round lower part
plus
hinges
and lower cast
with
heel cup
support brace
and controls
lower fragment
rotation

(a)

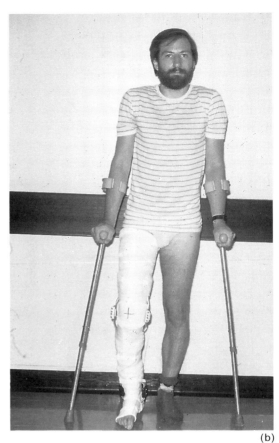

(b)

Figure 10.10 *a* A schematic representation of a femoral
cast brace. *b* An early Sheffield system brace built on the
principles illustrated in *a*. Note how a strip of material, *c*,
may be removed to make the brace adjustable.

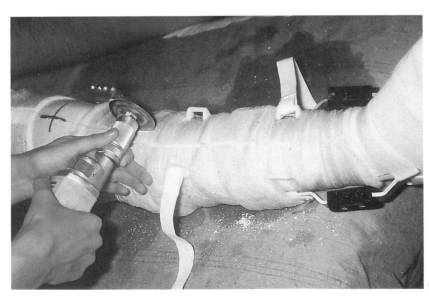

(c)

not the fracture—and confer rotatory control on the distal femoral fracture fragment.

Points to be watched in construction are:

1. To ensure that the brace reaches to the greater trochanter laterally but does not impinge on the ischium postero-medially—a brace is not an ischial-bearing device.

2. The fit of the femoral cuff must be accurate and no padding should be placed on this component. For this reason it is desirable to build the brace on a shaped cotton sock that affords adequate protection and provides a firm foundation for the brace.

3. The hinges should be applied using a jig to ensure that they are accurately placed, central to the patella and two-thirds of the way back.

4. The lower component should be snug without being tight and may be lightly padded. The brace should stop just above the malleoli to prevent rubbing if an ankle hinge is to be used.

5. If a plastic ankle cup is used, it should be made removable to avoid skin excoriation.

A polyurethane brace once set, after an hour, can be cut anteriorly and a strip removed without affecting the integrity of the rest of the structure. This may be done above and below the knee. The brace can then be made adjustable by means of Velcro straps held in place by double-sided tape. The success of this type of brace in Sheffield has led to the development of special clasps that can be incorporated into the material during construction. These are particularly advantageous for the elderly and infirm of hand (Figure 10.11).

The tibial brace (Figure 10.12)

Sarmiento first designed his patellar-bearing cast as a bucket-like structure in which the limb was suspended exactly as in a below-knee prosthesis for an amputee. As already explained, we now know that the brace works by a much more subtle mechanism. Sarmiento still retains his boss around the femoral condyles in his preformed braces and claims that it aids in rotatory control in flexion by remaining in contact with the femoral condyles. However, a close examination of an average brace fails to bear out this observation as the boss usually sits proud of the femur and serves no function. In addition, Sarmiento's own figures[20] demonstrate no significant improvement in rotatory

Figure 10.11 Large and small clasps which can be incorporated into polyurethane to make adjustment easier. Their use is illustrated in Figure 10.14.

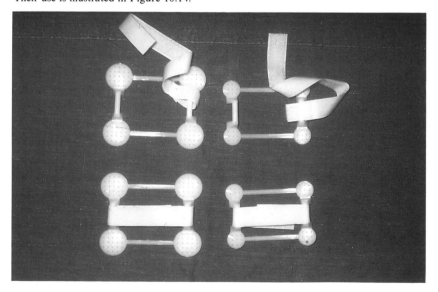

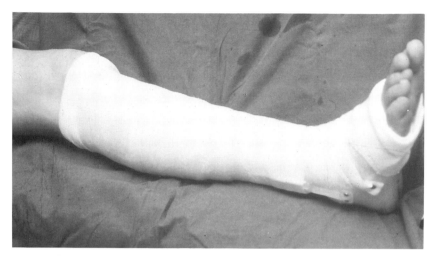

Figure 10.12 A simple tibial brace without an
adjustment slit. This should be fashioned once the brace
has set but before the patient is discharged. The absence of
a patellar boss is discussed in the text.

Figure 10.13 A simple humeral brace during
construction. Note how the stockinette is doubled so that
the outer layer, adherent to the polyurethane, will slide
over the inner sleeve during adjustment. The adjusters will
be added and the slit cut one hour later when the material
has consolidated its lamination through chemical setting.

control when the femoral boss is added. For simplicity, therefore, the boss may be omitted but it is
essential to ensure that the fit of the upper third of the
brace is intimate around the tibial tubercle and that it
is slightly flattened at the back against the soft tissues
so as to give a triangular profile.

For adjustment, a cut at the front seems to be as
satisfactory as a slit at the back, and no overlap is
required to prevent sharp edges digging into the pliant
calf. In an unpublished series of over fifty tibial
fractures treated in this way in Sheffield, there has
been no incidence of excessive anterior or posterior
bowing owing to an anterior slit position.

The humeral brace (Figure 10.13)

There is nothing simpler than the construction of a
humeral brace using polyurethanes, and providing a
few points are watched this is a very satisfactory way
of treating humeral shaft fractures.

1. The arm must be relaxed, as hunching of the
shoulder will result in the brace being applied with
the distal fragment in varus. For similar reasons, the
elbow should be at an angle of 90 degrees. The
optimal position is with the patient sitting and

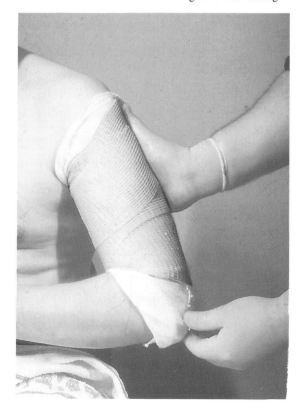

nursing his or her affected elbow at a right angle across the lap, supported by the unaffected hand.

2. The brace functions in conjunction with a collar and cuff sling which permits the arm to lie gently alongside the chest in neutral rotation. A sling higher than a right angle will cause a varus deformity.

The forearm brace (Figure 10.14)

This brace is designed solely for the treatment of isolated ulnar injuries and must not be confused with the more complex radius and ulnar brace. It consists of a simple cylinder around the forearm. It is adjustable and if maintained snug will permit normal, non-load-bearing function of the forearm. It may be used in the early stages in conjunction with a triangular bandage, but patients soon gain sufficient confidence to make reasonable use of their arm.

The destroyed elbow brace
(Figure 10.15)

Duckworth points out that one of the contraindications to internal fixation of fractures is that fixation may not be feasible.[21] A good example of this is the grossly disrupted elbow, particularly in the elderly, where bone quality is poor. In this small but significant group of patients an acceptable alternative to surgery is early mobilization even in the face of grossly disordered anatomy. A full arm brace incorporating an elbow hinge is a useful adjuvant to this line of management. A little care is required to ensure accurate hinge alignment as no jig is available. One of the advantages of the Sheffield type of hinge is that the available window of axis will accommodate small errors.

This brace can also be used for the rare cases where a pathological fracture cannot be fixed. Although internal fixation is the first line of management of pathological fractures around the elbow, the bracing method at least serves to illustrate how pathological fractures do unite, providing the site has been irradiated.

Figure 10.14 A forearm brace with two Sheffield Masterclasps in position making the finished product adjustable but not easily removable.

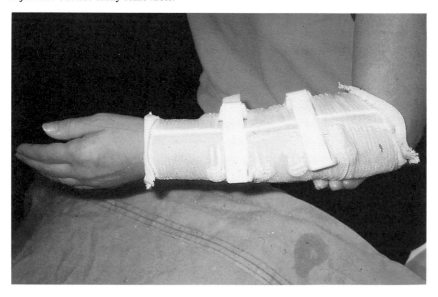

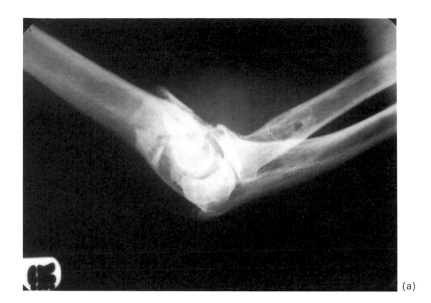

(a)

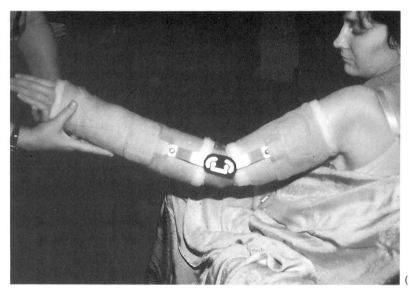

(b)

Figure 10.15 *a* A grossly disrupted elbow: internal
fixation, if feasible at all, would be fraught with hazard. *b*
A simple full arm brace using a small Sheffield hinge. This
brace need not be adjustable if swelling is not gross
because its role is to align the joint rather than bones
within soft tissues.

Pre- and post-bracing management

Before the brace

Most errors of management and poor results from bracing have their foundation in the early treatment period. When braces are blamed for late loss of position the problem can often be traced back to poor position in the pre-bracing phase and subsequent malposition at the time of bracing. Sarmiento has shown that fractures do not shorten from the position observed just before bracing and the same applies, although not to quite the same extent, to angulation. It must be accepted that late angulation occurs, but this may be attributed to other factors such as an intact fellow bone, too high a fracture or simply bad brace fitting. If all the rules have been obeyed, late positional losses are rare.

Most patients are treated on traction before bracing of the lower limb. This is undoubtedly the most difficult technique of fracture treatment in general use today. It requires constant vigilance from medical and nursing staff if positions are to be maintained. Skeletal traction is easier to manage than the adhesive method. Static traction is advisable if the nursing and junior doctor support is inexpert, provided it is not to be maintained for more than two or three weeks. Sliding or balanced traction is preferred if expert supervision is available because in this way movement is initiated early.

Many of the difficulties of traction are caused at the very beginning of treatment. It is a holding technique, very much dependent on the muscles surrounding the fracture moulding the bones together by their tone, which is in turn stimulated by the weights. It is not sufficient to find a rough position at initial reduction and hope the traction will do the rest. Radiographs should be taken with the patient in bed and still under anaesthetic. It is then possible to get the traction right at the outset and much awkward and possibly futile adjustment will be avoided. If the position cannot be consistently maintained by traction, soft tissue support immediately around the fracture may be deficient and loss of subsequent position in the brace is more likely.

The timing of brace application

There can be no hard and fast rule as to when a brace should be applied except that it should be put on as soon as possible. Again we must turn to fundamental research from Sarmiento suggesting that a fracture treated in a 'functional environment' will develop a local blood supply superior to that of a fracture treated by prolonged immobilization. Kenwright et al., examining the effects of axial motion through an external fixator, show that fracture stiffness is accelerated in the presence of micromovement.[22] It would appear that these effects are not seen initially for the first few weeks following injury and there is no advantage from very early bracing.

A frequently expressed opinion is that bracing should be reserved until the fracture is 'sticky'. This is an odd term because fractures do not stiffen in a progressive, linear fashion, but in steps. Thus a very mobile fracture one day may be quite stiff the next, and occasionally vice versa.[23] To await for an imagined 'stickiness' is to betray a lack of confidence in brace construction and to misconceive brace function.

In practice, bracing before three weeks seems of little value to the fracture and because of swelling may result in the brace having to be reapplied. Too early bracing may be painful, so providing the patient with no advantage in mobility, and it may result in his losing confidence in the brace early on in treatment. Bracing of an average fracture after six weeks brings little advantage in the way of intrinsic healing through blood supply. However, a late brace could help to mobilize the patient early, perhaps even allowing him to get back to sedentary employment. Most bracing should therefore be carried out not earlier than two to three weeks and preferably not after six weeks. The later end of the spectrum should be reserved for the higher velocity injuries when soft tissue damage has been more extensive. The economic advantages of bracing include savings in bed occupancy and even in transport costs as the patient wearing a brace may be able to use public transport to and from hopspital instead of expensive ambulances.

After the brace

The patient should have a check radiograph immediately after the brace is applied and then be seen within a few days, or detained in hospital until weight-bearing is established. In lower limb fractures weight-bearing with the aid of crutches should be encouraged as soon as possible. A check radiograph at a few days is advisable to ensure there is no positional loss, and at the same time the brace can be checked for fit.

The patient should be instructed on how to look after the brace and to keep the fit snug. The full brace should initially be worn continuously. A detachable heel cup may be removed at night later on and instructions given for daily cleansing of the foot under the cup. If a non-porous material is used, the patient may need to attend the hospital for skin maintenance; as mentioned, a great advantage of the glass fibre and polyurethane brace is that the underlying skin needs little attention during treatment.

Medical follow-up must include initial weekly radiographs for two weeks followed by monthly visits until union occurs. This will vary depending on the severity of the initial injury but should be between twelve and sixteen weeks in the lower limb and four to six weeks in the upper limb. The decision to remove the brace is based on the radiological features supported by physical examination. It is common and sensible to err on the side of caution and brace for slightly longer if there is any doubt.

Complications

The key to good management is to realize the limitations of the technique and be prepared to abandon it should serious problems arise. One of the great merits of functional bracing is that it is easy to do this. The principal problems likely to arise are:

Late loss of position

This so-called late loss of position can usually be attributed to poor pre-bracing managements, described earlier. Although termed 'late', indications that it may happen usually occur within a week or two of the brace being applied. Loss of position is difficult to correct by bracing and unless the fit has been very poor it is usually a sign that the fracture should be treated by other means.

Joint swelling

All the usual problems of applying a constricting structure to a limb pertain, and the patient should be warned to report any excessive pain, swelling, discoloration or change in sensation. These problems will be rare unless bracing is premature.

Swelling of the knee is common in femoral braces, particularly if they are not adjustable. It often causes alarm but in the author's experience it is of little significance providing it is not gross, or prejudicing the circulation. Knee swelling tends to disperse spontaneously when the brace is removed and there appear to be no long term sequelae.

Skin sores

Bracing should be avoided in the presence of skin

blisters and open wounds. Even without these lesions, a poorly fitting brace, particularly one made of a water impervious material, may rub. Patients' complaints of rubbing or burning of the skin must be taken seriously and the brace removed to check.

Contraindications to bracing

Among the fracture types discussed above there are a few not suitable for bracing. The upper third of the femur, the upper humerus and the grossly displaced tibial plateau must be avoided. Most dissatisfaction with bracing does not, however, arise from poor fracture selection but rather as a result of choosing unsuitable patients. Often braces are tried when all other methods have failed. When the brace also fails the method itself is condemned.

There are certain specific groups who are unsuitable for bracing. Confused, uncooperative and psychiatrically disturbed subjects should not be braced since this is a technique requiring rapport between clinician and patient. Patients with peripheral neuropathies are at severe risk of skin problems; these include all tablet- and insulin-dependent diabetics. The newcomer would be advised to avoid all such patients until he or she is experienced in the technique. Patients with peripheral vascular disease sufficient to result in loss of distal pulses should not be braced.

The future

Bracing is not a universal panacea even for the fracture groups that particularly lend themselves to the technique. The recent improvements in technology have reduced the initial period of learning and overcome many of the skill barriers that have limited the scope of functional bracing. Preformed braces seem to have a role, although they are not yet as adaptable as the manufacturers would have us believe, and they are certainly too expensive for widespread use. The preformed brace using new plastics and composites does offer an exciting future and will eventually become the most popular.

Increasing sophistication in hinge design, which permits physiological joint motion, has opened up new possibilities for the use of braces in soft tissue injuries. In particular, the hinges allow control of ranges of joint motion, and they are now being used to encourage high quality ligamentous repair. Braces as joint off-loading devices are being experimented with in the treatment of such conditions as Perthe's disease and even inoperable osteoarthrosis. So widespread are these developments that it is possible to ask, 'When is a brace not a brace and when does it become an orthosis?' The answer may be that these represent different ends of a spectrum that has been modified by developments in bracing rather than in the orthotic field. Unless attitudes to orthotics change, the proponents of bracing may fundamentally alter the approach to orthoses and calipers in the disabled, leaving the orthotist still using materials such as steel and leather, which in this field will be regarded as antediluvian within the next decade.

Interlocking medullary nailing

T. D. Bunker, BSc, MB, BS, MCh Orth,
FRCS, FRCS Ed

One man stands like a colossus over the history of medullary nailing; his name is Gerhardt Küntscher. His achievements span thirty years from his first medullary nailing in 1939 to his description of detensor nailing (interlocking nailing) in 1968.

The last decade has seen the development of interlocking nailing extending the potential of medullary nailing to areas of the long bones that were hitherto technically impossible to nail. This potential is not yet fully developed.

History

The first primitive attempts at medullary fixation were probably performed by Heine in 1875 using ivory pegs.[1] In 1889 Senn, of Milwaukee, used a nail of aseptic iron driven up the femoral neck and achieved bony union of a femoral neck fracture.[2] Lillienthal in 1910 used an aluminium medullary splint on a compound infra-isthmal fracture of the femur, at Bellevue Hospital, New York.[3]

At the same time, in Britain, Hey Groves started his experimental work on medullary nailing. He compared various materials—ivory, bone, aluminium and steel. He also experimented on a cat with an absorbable nail made of magnesium, which disappeared from the femur within three weeks.[4] Realizing that short bone pegs, although opposing the bone ends did not create sufficient immobility of the fracture ends, he started to invent different ways of inserting longer

nails. His first effort was to produce a nail with a transverse drill hole at the mid-point of its length. A loop of wire was inserted through this hole and the nail was driven from the fracture site up the medullary canal until it disappeared, leaving only the loop of wire coming out of the bone (Figure 11.1). The fracture was then reduced and the wire loop retrieved using a special wire-tightening device. In the process, the nail was gradually pulled out of the proximal fragment into the distal fragment. It was a short step from this to pushing a longer nail out through the trochanter, and then hammering this back down into the distal fragment: the retrograde method of nailing described by Hey Groves in 1916. He used pegs of various shapes, cylindrical, cruciform (Figure 11.2) and solid rods. These last he believed to be the best. He described four cases of septic and non-septic non-union of the femur treated by medullary nailing.[5] He concluded that the 'long internal peg' was 'one of some value in special cases'. In his Bradshaw Lecture to the Royal College of Surgeons in 1926[6] he stated (on nailing femoral neck fractures), 'I think the operation should be done under the guidance of the fluorescent screen'—showing again his remarkable foresight.

Advances in medullary fixation have often gone hand in hand with developments in materials, and so it was that Müller-Meernach in 1933 reported on 26 cases treated by pinning with round or cross-shaped pins made of rust-free Krupp steel.[7]

At this time Küntscher was working at the Kiel Surgical Clinic on 'the callus problem'. He was

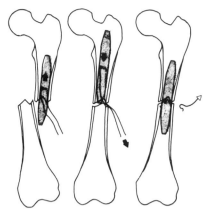

Figure 11.1 The Hey Groves 'long peg', showing its method of insertion.

Figure 11.2 The Hey Groves original nail.

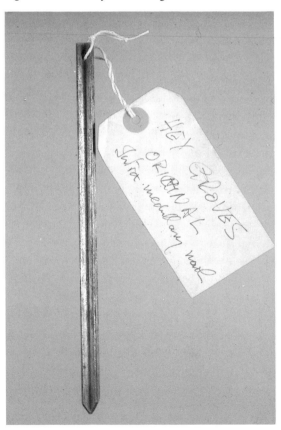

fascinated to discover that he could incite a callus response without fracture using rusting iron wire in the dog tibia,[8] and yet femoral neck fractures healed without callus. So he came to know of Müller-Meernach's work. Küntscher took a cannulated Smith-Petersen nail and had the idea of turning this around into the femoral canal. Next, using a V profile nail made of corrosion free V2A steel, he nailed a subtrochanteric femoral fracture in 1939. He presented his method to the German Surgical Society, commenting that its advantage would be of great benefit in time of war.[9]

Work by inexperienced surgeons in the field could not have been as successful as that emanating from Kiel, for in 1942 Küntscher found himself posted to Kemmi, in Finnish Lapland, just south of the Arctic Circle, until 1944 when the army withdrew. From 1946 Küntscher worked at Schleswig Hesterberg near the Danish border under extremely difficult conditions. Despite this and his lack of university backing, he further developed his percutaneous method under image intensifier control.

In 1957, Küntscher moved to the Hafen Hospital in Hamburg, until his retirement in 1965. In 1968, he reported the use of transverse screws at the top and bottom of the nail in comminuted fractures (Figure 11.3) to prevent shortening and rotation of the fracture. He termed this the 'detensing effect'. In 1970, Klemm took up the detensing idea for infected pseudarthroses and then for comminuted fractures. With Küntscher's approval he changed the name from detensing to interlocking. Küntscher died in 1972 while writing a further edition of his book on medullary nailing.

Others had been working on the interlocking principles during this period. In 1940 in Russia, Fishkin used a nail deploying fins to compress a femoral shaft fracture. In 1953 in the United States, Modny[10] developed a perforated cruciate nail with cross screws to prevent migration. Thus we have three schools of interlocking nails: those based on Küntscher's detensor, the Klemm, Grosse-Kempf, AO and Richards' nails; those based on Fishkin's, deploying fins, the Brooker-Wills and Derby nails; and those similar to Modny's nail, the compression nail of Huckstep.

It is only right that this chapter should be based on Küntscher's four principles of fracture fixation, together with discussion of their application in the interlocking era. These are:

1. Fixation of the fragments so they will not part

2. Closed nailing

3. Favourable conditions for callus formation

4. Simplicity.

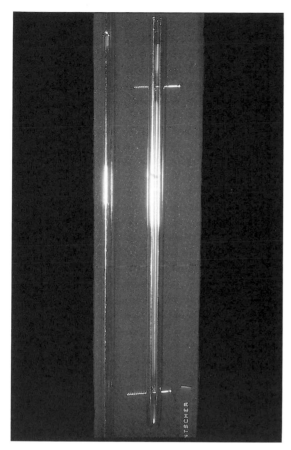

Figure 11.3 Küntscher's 'detensing nail'.

The BS conversion, by its practical application, should make the theory more comprehensible.[11] The BS conversion is the force required to break a broomstick, which is 45 Newton metres. To break a broomstick, a bending, or angular force of 45 Newtons must be applied 1 metre from the centre of rotation (in this case the site of fracture). This is termed a *moment*, and is measured in Newton metres.

The bending force to break the average adult femur is 250 Newton metres. In other words, a femur is six times as strong as a broomstick.

Bending rigidity is proportional to the cube of the thickness of the medullary nail (in the direction of the loading force). A medullary nail of double thickness has its bending rigidity increased by a factor of 8. Thus a small change in the diameter of the nail can improve bending strength greatly.

Working length The problem for a medullary nail is that rigidity is inversely proportional to the cube of the working length. This is not the length of the rod but the length between the two main points where the bone has purchase on the rod. Thus, for a short, oblique fracture fixed by a well fitting rod in a reamed canal, the working length is small, the rigidity high. However, a comminuted fracture fixed by an interlocking nail has a long working length with low rigidity (Figure 11.4).

Fixation of the fragments so that they will not part

The orthopaedic surgeon performing a medullary nailing creates a new structure from the wreckage of the old. In so doing he becomes a structural engineer. It is, therefore, important that he understands some basic engineering principles, so that by choosing the structure of his implant he may solve his fracture problems. This has become increasingly important with the proliferation of interlocking nails.

Brief definitions of the major biomechanical terms should be helpful for non-engineers:

Force is a product of mass and acceleration ($F = m \times a$). It is measured in Newtons (the force required to accelerate a mass of 1 Kg at 1 m/sec^2).

Figure 11.4 Working lengths: *left*, a short working length produces a more rigid nail-bone construct than, *right*, a long working length.

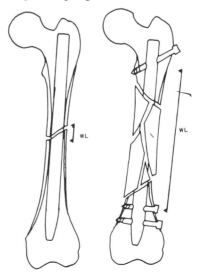

Torsional rigidity increases with the 4th power of the radius of the nail. Doubling the radius of a solid rod increases rigidity by 16 times. This torsional rigidity still has to be imparted from the nail to the fracture and this will depend on the area of contact between the nail and the bone; this is increased by reaming and having a snug fitting elastic nail. The other means of transmitting the torsional rigidity to the fracture is by interlock.

Open section

Most medullary nails have a slot along their length to give elastic fixation along the reamed medullary canal, so as to impart torsional rigidity. Such is the trade-off that this slot reduces the torsional rigidity of the nail by 5 to 6 times. This is especially significant in interlocking nails of increased working length (q.v.). Since interlocking nails do not need elastic fixation against the medullary canal to transmit their torsional rigidity (indeed in long comminuted fractures there may be no canal), they can be made more rigid by being constructed of a closed section (Richards' nail, Derby nail, new Grosse-Kempf nail).

Nail shape

Rigidity can be altered 5 to 6 times by altering the cross-sectional shape of the nail in the direction of the loading force. For the same mass of material a cylinder is stronger than a solid rod. (This is not to say that a cylinder is stronger than a rod of the same diameter, for a rod of the same diameter must have a greatly increased mass.) In terms of strength in all directions, for its mass, the cylinder is the best and this is why nature has selected it for the construction of our long bones. Most medullary nails follow nature's pattern.

Let us now consider the principles of fixation. The nailed femur must keep the bone fragments together. This means that it must resist the forces placed upon it by gravity, muscle pull and normal conditions of use during rehabilitation, until the bone has regained its former strength.

The major muscle groups acting on the fractured femur depend on the level of fracture. In upper third fractures the main deforming muscle pulls are of the abductors on the greater trochanter, and of iliopsoas on the lesser trochanter. These displace the proximal fragment into abduction and flexion, causing a varus deformity (Figure 11.5).

In middle third fractures the deforming forces are the pull of the adductors, causing a varus deformity, along with gravity on the lower leg and foot causing

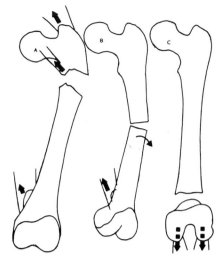

Figure 11.5 The usual patterns of malunion of femoral fracture: *a* a high fracture will flex the proximal fragment. *b* A midshaft fracture will go into varus and external rotation. *c* A low fracture will cause extension of the distal fragment.

an external rotation deformity. Lower third fractures are pulled into extension by the pull of gastrocnemius.

The normal conditions that the femur must withstand during rehabilitation, including walking, amount to one half the force required to fracture it, that is, 125 Newton metres. The smallest AO nail that can withstand this force is 13 mm. Thus, for an average adult male 13 mm is the minimum nail diameter.

Failure

Mechanical failure of the nail occurs in one of two ways—plastic deformation or fatigue failure. If the nail is overloaded it passes its yield point and deforms. The nail should be changed for one with a wider diameter. Fatigue failure usually occurs at a stress riser. Any hole, sharp angle, notch or groove in a structure produces a stress concentration effect, or stress riser. Two examples of stress risers in medullary nails were the junction between the open and closed section of the original AO medullary nails, which have been recorded as causing fatigue failures; and in the original Grosse-Kempf nail, the lower of the two proximal locking screw holes was placed too close to the open section of the nail, sometimes causing fatigue failure at this point. Both these problems have been eliminated with changes in the design of the nails.

Bending stability has been measured for most nails, and as long as a sufficient nail diameter is used, plastic deformation does not occur. This is not to say that there is no angular deformity as the nail may be introduced into the trochanter incorrectly (too laterally or too medially), or the nail may be sited eccentrically in the intercondylar notch.

It has been thought that a varus deformity is a greater menace to the knee than a valgus deformity.[12] However, Koostra[13] showed that although 41 per cent of patients treated on traction and 20 per cent of nailed patients had an angular deformity, none had symptoms related to angulation.

Rotational and compressive stability are therefore the most important potential reasons for the bone fragments parting. The hip allows for some correction of rotational deformity, but external rotation in excess of 20 degrees may cause degenerative arthritis of the lateral compartment of the knee.[12] Müller[14] felt that rotation could give rise to symptoms in the ankle and foot. In Koostra's vast veries,[13] a rotational deformity was found in 37 per cent of conservatively managed femurs and, surprisingly, in 48 per cent of nailed femurs. This high incidence of rotation occurred postoperatively. Comparisons are of little value between series in the literature as the types of fracture pattern are so different, but it should be noted that in Winquist's series of 520 cases (closed femoral nailing), rotational deformity of greater than 20 degrees was seen in only 2.3 per cent (comminuted fractures were interlocked towards the end of the series).[15]

Biomechanically interlock seems to solve the rotational problem, so long as the rotation is correct at operation. Grosse-Kempf,[16] Brooker-Wills[17] and Derby[18] nails all show a fully elastic torsional stress/strain curve to 40 degrees of deflection, that is, they all 'spring back' to their original configuration when the torsional load is removed. Consequently 89 per cent of Brooker-Wills interlocked fractures had less than 10 degrees' rotational deformity,[19] and even with severe comminution 84 per cent of Grosse-Kempf interlocked fractures had less than a 5 degrees' rotational deformity.[20]

There remains the problem of shortening. Shortening in excess of 2 cm leads to a disturbed walking pattern.[21] Late effects of shortening may be an equinus foot, compensatory scoliosis and low back pain.[12] Shortening of more than 4 cm is looked upon as a 15 per cent disability allowance in Sweden[22] and Germany.[12] Shortening in conservatively treated patients varies from 18 per cent[23] to 53 per cent[13] (shortening of at least 2 cm). This is reduced in all series of medullary nailing. Shortening of at least 2 cm in nailed series varies from 2 per cent,[15,19] to 3 per cent.[23,24] Even with severe comminution,[20] 11 per cent had shortening and all of these were early in the Grosse-Kempf series, more care being taken to correct length later in the study. Thus, operative treatment generally results in insignificant shortening, whereas conservative treatment frequently results in shortening, although this is usually slight.

Closed nailing

Küntscher firmly believed in healing of the incision as far away from the fracture as possible, the main reasons being a decrease in the rate of deep infection in unexposed fractures, and that the fracture haematoma is neither disturbed nor removed.

Closed nailing is dependent on a traction table, an image intensifier and a team (surgeon, unscrubbed assistant, radiographer and scrub nurse) who are experienced at the technique (Figure 11.6).

All authorities agree that preoperatively skeletal traction using a large load (up to 18 kg for an adult man) is essential to hold the fracture out to length, or, if possible, distract it. The timing of surgery is controversial. Many believe that there should be a delay of five to seven days before nailing, as this has been shown to secure a higher rate of union, and the risk of fat embolus syndrome has by that time passed.[25,26]

However, in major trauma centres there is a swing towards immediate closed nailing for multiply injured patients. This improves pulmonary function, aids chest physiotherapy and nursing care, leading to decreased morbidity.[27]

Open fractures are best treated initially on skeletal traction until the wound is cleanly granulating and the surgeon is satisfied that there is no evidence of infection. However, Winquist et al[15] have shifted to immediate closed nailing of Types I and II open femoral fractures. The wound is thoroughly debrided and left open. The deep infection rate in this study of 520 closed nailings is 0.9 per cent. It should be pointed out that this is the best result in the world literature, from a unit with a vast experience of the technique, and they changed their policy towards open fractures only late in their series.

Traction

At Nottingham the lateral position on the fracture table is used, with the hip and knee flexed. A perineal bar is essential and a tensioned Kirschner wire is inserted across the femoral condyles for distraction.

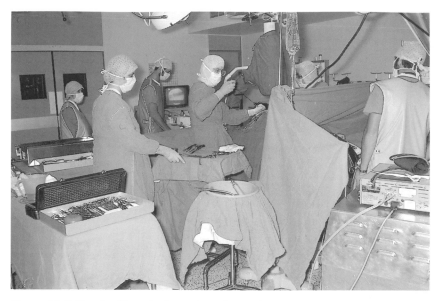

Figure 11.6 Closed nailing of a femur depends on a team of surgeons, anaesthetists, nurses and radiographers.

The perineal bar, and particularly its upward extension can give rise to problems. Pressure upon the bar can cause perineal oedema, and pudendal nerve palsy.[28] Pressure sores have even been known. Pressure on the femoral vein may cause a high venous pressure preoperatively, with increased bleeding at interlock sites, or at the fracture site in the rare instances when it has to be exposed. Pressure on the femoral artery will cause a mottled discoloration of the foot, which must be looked for when traction is applied; this is reversible when traction is removed. The conclusion is that forceful distraction is required during closed nailing. Since this is not without problems, the traction should be released as soon as possible.

The traction wire across the femoral condyles should be placed posterior to the midline of the femur, otherwise it lies directly where the nail tip should come to rest. It is not unknown for the last seating down of the nail to bend the wire, making it extremely difficult to remove. In at least one case[29] it was impossible to remove the bent, incarcerated traction wire, which had to be cut off below the skin; a somewhat embarrassing situation for patient and surgeon alike.

Before the patient is prepared, the unscrubbed assistant checks that reduction is possible, and the radiographer that his C arm travel gives good views of the fracture in both directions. Fresh fractures tend to align themselves quite easily with traction alone, but the greater the delay, the more difficult the reduction. The reduction is performed by the unscrubbed assistant using a lead gloved hand, wooden wrench, crutch and sling or, best of all, circular reduction rings (Figure 11.7).

At Nottingham, the patient is draped using a clear plastic hip exclusion drape which covers the whole body. Sterile covers are put on the image intensifier. The surgeon can also help in the reduction by putting a narrow (8 mm) Küntscher nail into the perforated greater trochanter and using it as a lever to swing the proximal fragment in line with the distal. Passing the guide wire is made easier by bending the tip 20 degrees and rotating the bent end into the distal fragments. The guide wire is passed to the intercondylar notch and is checked in two planes on the image intensifier.

Reaming and nail insertion

Reaming is then carried out to 0.5 mm greater than the required nail diameter. The guide wires are exchanged inside the wash tube, and the canal is washed out and sucked clean. The appropriate nail is

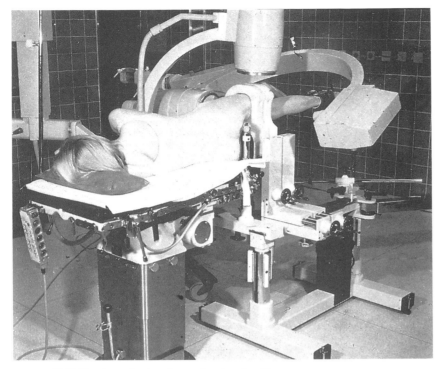

Figure 11.7 Circular reduction clamps for closed nailing.

then inserted. The fracture must be screened as the nail is passed, or it may catch on the distal fragment, leading to comminution. The Biomet 'pathfinder nails' have a bullet-shaped tip to prevent catching. Rotation should then be checked, and corrected if necessary.

Distal interlocking

For interlocking nails, the distal interlock is then performed. This is not easy. Everybody who has performed a large number of distal interlocks has a story to tell. Early interlocking nail designs had a distal interlocking jig which attached to the proximal, driving section, of the nail. Unfortunately open section nails can twist as they go down the curved femoral canal by up to 45 degrees. These jigs have been discontinued for open section nails, but the new Richards' nail, having a closed section, utilizes this type, as does the solid titanium Huckstep compression nail.

Grosse and Kempf tried a distal jig mounted to the

image intensifier, but many surgeons found this cumbersome and that the intensifier wobbled. Some surgeons reverted to the original Klemm distal interlock method of exposing a short section of distal femur, finding the screw holes on the intensifier and marking the bone at this point with an awl, or perforator. The screw holes could then be drilled.

The AO distal interlock has an ingenious system of concentric dots and circles to line up on the distal interlock holes. Even this is not without problems, however, as the jig is bulky and clashes with the Kirschner wire and traction bow.

Clearly, such problems with the distal interlock, which has to be performed under image intensifier control, lead to concern over the radiation dose to the patient and theatre personnel.

Radiation

Grosse measured the radiation dose during 30 interlocking procedures,[20] using direct reading dosimeters. It was found that exposure is insignificant at over 0.8

metres from the radiation source, if the image intensifier has an image store and if the distal targeting device is used. With a 0.5 mm lead apron body, exposure was unmeasurable. The image store reduced the radiation dose by 60 per cent. Average radiation time was 2 minutes 38 seconds for the reduction and 1 minute 4 seconds for the introduction of the nail and locking screws. Two comments should be made in relation to these comforting facts. First, many surgeons have given up the targeting devices and have to stand closer than 0.8 metres to the source during distal interlock. Second, these average times are for a unit that has performed over 400 interlocking nailings. In other units with little or no experience on the part of the radiographer or surgeon, radiation times could be expected to be higher. In Nottingham, a study was run using sterilizable ring dosimeters on the surgeons' index fingers. The screening time was longer than the Strasbourg series (Table 11.1) and yet the radiation dose was still acceptable (Table 11.2).

In an attempt to reduce the radiation dose, Klemm[30] has been using a set of target magnets with Hall effect transducers to locate the hole in the nail without X-ray imaging. It is hoped that this approach will prove successful.

The problems of the distal interlock are by no means solved. In order to get around the radiation problem, nails of the deploying fin type ascribed to Fishkin have been developed; in particular, the Brooker-Wills and Derby nails. In the Brooker-Wills type, the deploying fins are inserted down the centre of the nail, being guided by the clover-leaf shape of the nail (Figure 11.8). Deployment is checked under image intensifier control, but from a safe distance. In a series of 103 nails,[19] 3 had problems with deployment, owing to nail or fracture rotation.

The Derby nail has built-in deploying fins (Figure 11.9). These are opened by inserting a screw into the proximal nail. Deployment is watched under image intensifier control from outside the 0.8 metre line, and no problems were encountered in 22 pathological fractures.[31] The Derby nail is closed-sectioned, so there is no risk of nail rotation with it. However, owing to the inbuilt nature of the fins, the Derby nail

Table 11.1 Image intensifier screening times for three different centres (in minutes)

	Redn + Nail Prox Lock	Distal Lock	Total
Nottingham (N = 10)	5.56	6.52	12.08
Houston (N = 30)*	7.42	5.12	12.6
Strasbourg (N = 452)**	2.52	1.05	3.57

*Leuin et al 1987 *JBJS*
**Grosse & Kempf 1985 *JBJS*

Table 11.2 Radiation dosage during locking nailing

	dom	n/dom	neck	g/u	pt	ctrl
Mean dose equivalent mSv						
Nottingham	0.71	0.39	0.44	0.11	1.81	0.12
Houston (G—K)	0.25	—	0.15	—	—	—
Acceptable yearly dose equ. mSv	300	300	300	50	5	50

(Reproduced from *Injury* by permission of the publishers, Butterworth & Co [Publishers] Ltd)

Figure 11.8 The deploying fins of the Brooker-Wills nail.

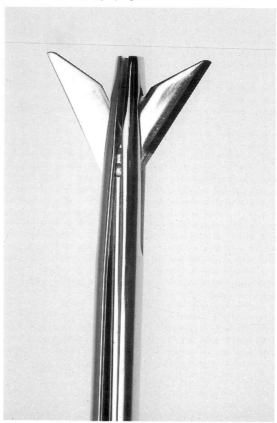

the medullary canal. Fortunately theory and practice do not coincide in this instance. Callus does generally form, rates of delayed and non-union are low, and although radiological union may take some months, in the most recent series these patients are walking from the third post-operative day.[19,20]

It is an undisputed fact that medullary reaming and tight nailing destroy the marrow, nutrient arteries and their main and small branches. However, vessels survive in the richly vascular metaphyses as well as in the periosteal and extraosseous tissues.

The immediate effect of this destruction is extensive cortical ischaemia and necrosis. Rhinelander has shown experimentally in the dog[32] cortical necrosis of one-half to two-thirds of the cortex in areas of intimate contact between the nail and the bone; where the nail was loose, medullary circulation was rapidly restored. This may have relevance to a new generation of thinner, closed-section interlocking nails where reaming and elastic medullary fit are not so important. In man, cortical necrosis is extensive,[33] but loss of osteocytes is often incomplete and sometimes patchy.

The patchy nature of osteocyte death in man, along with the thrombi and fat droplet artefacts in Haversian canals indicate that other factors are at work.[34]

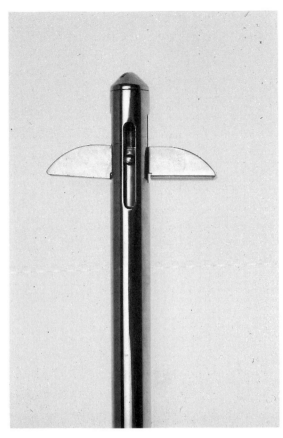

Figure 11.9 The deploying fins of the Derby nail.

is not cannulated and thus has to be inserted under screening after removal of the guide wire.

In contrast, the proximal interlock does not appear to have great problems, most jigs being satisfactory.

Favourable conditions for callus formation

Küntscher's third principle of medullary nailing was that conditions should be suitable for callus formation. Now, medullary nailing is theoretically unsound, for the nail necessarily destroys the medullary circulation. Reaming is theoretically even worse, causing complete medullary vascular destruction and heat necrosis, producing fat and debris to clog local and distant vessels and generating high pressures in

Embolization

Dankwart Lilliestrom[34] used marrow suction in the experimental animal to reduce embolization of fat and marrow. Marrow suction reduced cortical necrosis, suggesting that cortical perfusion was rapidly restored by reversal of the usual efferent (centrifugal) cortical blood flow. Unfortunately Rhinelander also used marrow suction and yet most of the cortex became necrotic. Results of marrow suction in man are unknown. External osteogenesis was reduced by marrow suction showing the osteogenic potential of the reamings. This was a reasonable trade-off, for in the group of rabbits undergoing marrow suction before identical nailing of a standard tibial osteotomy, there was a lesser degree of cortical damage, rapid bone formation in the fracture gap and remodelling. In the group that did not have bone marrow suction, there was greater cortical damage, slower revascularization of the cortex and resorption of the avascular fracture ends. Cortical resorption was so great that the nails often became loose before the callus had stabilized the fracture, and there was marked soft tissue swelling and eventually more callus. Bone healing was both superior and more rapid in the rabbits in the marrow suction group.

The heat of reaming may also cause cortical necrosis, and temperatures up to 50°C have been recorded during reaming of sheep tibiae. This heat depends on reamer sharpness, speed, pressure and cooling with saline.

High medullary pressures have been recorded during reaming. Pressures of 800 mmHg to 1500 mmHg have been demonstrated in sheep tibiae with medullary tissues being forced out under the periosteum.

Perhaps the ideal would be to perform medullary suction before and after reaming with the filtered-off reamings being replaced in the fracture haematoma under sterile conditions after nailing.

Revascularization

The next phase in the healing of medullary nailed fractures is revascularization. This occurs from extraosseous, cortical, metaphyseal and periosteal vessels. Many elegant experiments have shown that neither metaphyseal nor periosteal vessels are essential for healing, but extraosseous vessels and cortical vessels are. The surrounding muscles and soft tissues become hyperaemic and migrating vessels are accompanied by fibroblasts, osteogenic and mesenchymal cells. The cortex becomes more vascular, with resorptive widening of bone canals and cortical osteoporosis. Subperiosteal osteogenesis occurs, producing callus (Figure 11.10).

Early weight-bearing

Yamagishi and Yoshimura[35] showed that compression loading promoted healing of transverse tibial osteotomies. Panjabi[36] showed that initial compressive load followed by later cyclical loading favoured healing. Goodship[37] has shown increased fracture stiffness and greater callus production with cyclical loading of sheep tibial osteotomies.

These experimental findings lead us to believe that early weight-bearing should speed fracture healing. This is the aim of medullary nailing. Winquist achieved partial weight-bearing at an average of three days post-operatively,[15] the Derby group full weight-bearing in pathological fractures at 3 days,[31] and in severe comminuted fractures Grosse achieved crutch walking, non-weight-bearing, at three days.[20] This can be compared to Thomas and Meggit's average stay *in bed* for conservative treatment of 92 days.[38] In our series of AO interlocking nails from Nottingham, for isolated femoral fractures we had a hospital stay of 16 days, compared to Winquist's 13 days (B. J. Holdsworth, personal communication, 1986).

The snag with interlocking nails is that although the patient can be rapidly mobilized, the fracture is

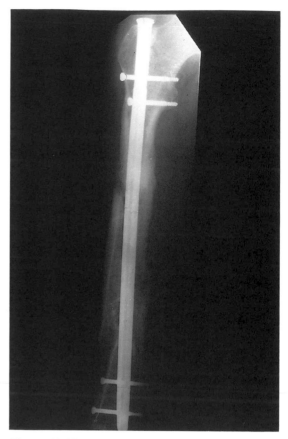

Figure 11.10 Callus following closed locking nailing.

actually *unloaded*. The nail becomes a weight-bearing device (Figure 11.11), instead of the ideal weight-sharing device, and thus bone union will be delayed.

Interlocking nails with deploying fins allow some controlled compression and are thus a partial weight-sharing/bearing device. The AO interlocking nail has a slotted proximal screw hole allowing some weight-sharing.

Fortunately, practice defies theory yet again, and interlocking nailed fractures appear to throw out good callus even when statically loaded. This may be a reflection of the different type of fracture for which interlocking nails are presently used: these are proximal or distal fractures with a rich metaphyseal blood supply, and midshaft comminuted fractures with a large fracture area. In our interlocking series, 52 per cent were comminuted fractures, and 42 per cent upper or lower third.

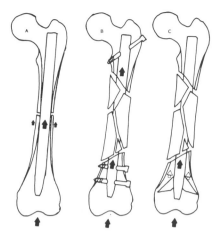

Figure 11.11 *Left*, the medullary nail is a weight-sharing device; *centre*, the statically locked nail is a weight-bearing device; *right*, the distal fin interlocking nail is weight-sharing.

Overall, mean time to consolidation in Grosse's series of comminuted fractures treated by Grosse-Kempf interlocking nail was 4.5 months. Brooker's series of fractures treated with his interlocking nail united at a mean time of 4.4 months, with one exception in 92 fractures. Although results from personal series by the originators of the nails are not always achievable in other hands, our early results on 50 patients followed for over six months using the AO interlocking nail are very good. Most were able to crouch, tiptoe and stand on their heels and had resumed work.

Simplicity

Simplicity was Küntscher's fourth principle. It has to be said that recent advances have diverged from it. Although closed nailing is relatively simple, it does rely on the complex machinery of the image intensifier with memory, the fracture table and powered flexible reamers.

Transverse screw distal interlocking cannot be described as simple, quick or radiation free; but perhaps deploying fin distal interlocking will simplify the procedure in the future.

Complications

Infection is the greatest worry of the surgeon performing medullary nailing. Although it can be kept to low levels (0.9 per cent for Winquist's 520 nailings), each infection is a disaster to the patient concerned. Scrupulous attention to detail, prophylactic antibiotics, medullary lavage and wound lavage using a closed procedure, all aim to reduce the infection rate. If infection does occur, reaming out the infected canal, washing and stabilization with a larger nail, followed by closed irrigation systems and long-term antibiotics should be applied in an attempt to control the situation.

Fat embolus syndrome remains a concern, with a rate of 10 per cent in Winquist's series and 13 per cent at Nottingham. However, a change to early nailing in Winquist's series did not increase the incidence of FES. It was therefore thought to be due to the fracture rather than the nailing procedure.

Perineal haematomas, pudendal nerve palsy, meralgia parasthetica and peroneal nerve palsy have all been reported secondary to high distraction forces.

Advantages and disadvantages

The advantages of interlocking nailing are increased stability in length and rotation, with maintenance of length even where there is severe comminution by closed methods. Compression is possible, allowing greater stability, early return to walking, early hospital discharge and return to work. Virtually all diaphyseal fractures can be dealt with, extending the scope of medullary nailing.

The disadvantages of the method are the possibility of infection, loss of the medullary blood supply, embolization caused by reaming, the need for a highly competent surgeon and an exceptional radiographer. It has also to be admitted that there are still difficulties attached to the distal interlocking procedure.

Each surgeon will have to balance these factors in his own mind, for each particular fracture, for each particular patient.

The ideal nail

So what is the ideal nail? Is it a cannulated, narrow closed-section, taper-ended nail contoured to the internal bowing and shape of the femur; strong enough to withstand 150 Newton metres of bending force, yet more pliable than metal; with deployable fin distal interlock giving full elastic springback to 40 degrees of torsion and proximal transverse screw jigged interlock; inserted closed into an unreamed medullary canal after marrow suction with injection of filtered, sterile, canal contents into the fracture haematoma under image intensifier control?

What of an absorbable nail, even? We come full circle to Hey Groves and his magnesium peg. I have presented the facts; I leave the reader to conjecture.

12

External fixation: past, present and future

A. G. MacEachern, MB, ChB, FRCS

The external fixator actually predates the plaster of Paris bandage by a decade. In 1843, Malgaigne[1,2] devised an external clamp to approximate transverse patellar fractures until healed (Figure 12.1). He saw two disadvantages in his device: first, the patients could remove the screw; second, in those preanaesthetic days, fitting of the fixator was very painful.

The Parkhill bone clamp,[3] with its four pins screwed into the bone, looked similar to some modern external fixators (Figure 12.2) and was adjustable in two directions. Parkhill was delighted with his results: all 14 tibial fractures united. Lambotte[4] devised a fixator which proved a great success. Its advantages in the management of fractures were that it could be rapidly and easily fitted, had great rigidity, allowed dressing of open wounds, removal was easy, and the limb could be actively and passively mobilized. Many of these qualities hold true to date.

In 1916, Hey Groves[5] documented his clinical experience in the human and his research ideas in the cat, involving treatment of long bone defects with external fixators.

In 1918, Crile[6] reported a case of a compound femoral fracture treated with his external fixator (Figure 12.3), describing for the first time the use of a universal ball joint, as well as a telescopic facility which offered the possibility of postoperative adjustment.

In the 1930s, external fixation of fractures was popularized mainly by the work of three people. The first was Anderson,[7] who devised a 'fracture robot' for the reduction of fractures, using transfixion pins

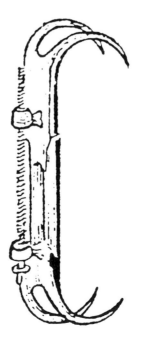

Figure 12.1 Malgaigne's claw, an external fixator for the patella (1843).

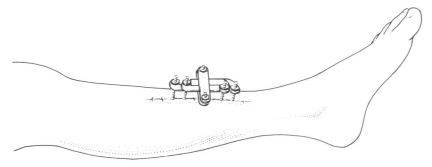

Figure 12.2 Parkhill's bone clamp. The first four-pin fixator with adjustment in two directions.

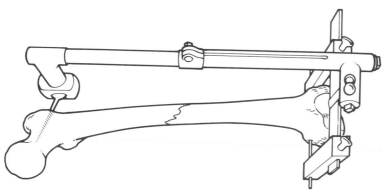

Figure 12.3 Crile's fixator, used in the First World War, has universal clamps for adjustment at each end.

connected to movable metal yokes. These allowed reduction of the fracture and compression before casting. He later eliminated the cast by connecting the pins with articulators to medial and lateral bars (Figure 12.4). Around that time, Stader,[8,9] a veterinary surgeon, developed an external fixator suitable for dogs. A larger version of this fixator was used by Lewis and Breidenbach[9] in humans. In 1938, Hoffman[10] described his unilateral fixator (Figure 12.5) with universal joints and a compressor/distractor.

Charnley[11] developed a method for compression arthrodesis of the knee,[8] and Judet[12] showed that compression could be useful in the management of pseudoarthroses (Figure 12.6). Vidal and his team[13] showed that extremely rigid fixation was required in septic non-union, and devised the quadrilateral Hoffman frame. However, Burny[14] continued to use the original Hoffman unilateral frame as an 'elastic

fixator'. In Russia, Ilisarov[15] and Volkov[16] developed ring fixators with thin transfixion wires.

The recent revival of external fixation is due to better understanding of pin tract sepsis, frame design and bone union.

Pin tract sepsis

This complication has prevented widespread acceptance of external fixation as a method of treating fractures other than the most complex. What is the magnitude of this problem compared to, for example, infection following the application of a diaphyseal plate? There has been little agreement between authors concerning the nature of pin tract infection. Burny[14] uses a standardized form for reporting the

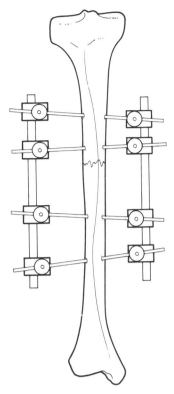

Figure 12.4 The Anderson frame, commonly used in the USA between the wars.

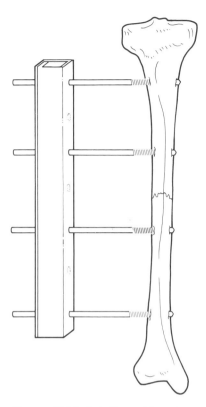

Figure 12.6 Judet's fixator (France).

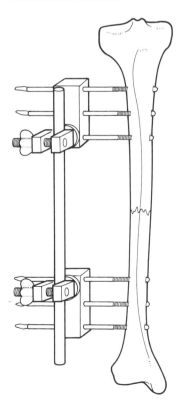

site and extent of sepsis, and has noted that, by 150 days, 10 per cent of pins develop signs of it; the rate increases sharply thereafter.

Green[17] introduced the concept of major and minor pin tract sepsis. A major infection involved hospital admission for parenteral antibiotics, pin removal or frame removal, and included chronic infection after pin removal. Any other, even purulent, reaction was classified as minor and required outpatient management. Green reviewed the literature and allocated the reported series to major and minor. He made two interesting observations: reported pin sepsis was lower in series using the pins in plaster technique (0.5 per cent), compared with external skeletal fixators

Figure 12.5 Hoffman's external fixator, the forebear of the present generation of unilateral fixators, adjustable in three dimensions (Switzerland).

(8.3 per cent). He also noted little change in the infection rate with time.

Recent research by Gie and MacEachern[18] attempts to classify pin sepsis into four categories (Table 12.1). Such a classification, if adopted, would allow better comparisons between different series.

Green[19] has eloquently described the pathophysiology of pin hole sepsis (see below).

Pin hole sepsis is the result of alteration in the balance between the host's defences and the infective capability of the bacteria. This may result from abscess formation around the pin; necrotic tissue

Figure 12.7 Motion and chemotaxis: *a* and *b* phagocytic whiteblood cell follows chemotactic gradient to bacterium; *c* white blood cell continues towards focus of gradient even if bacterium is moved away, until gradient becomes re-established in the opposite direction; *d* constant movement of milieu mixes gradient and reduces chemotactic efficiency.

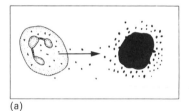

(a)

(b)

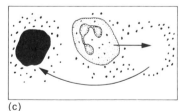

(c)

(d)

Table 12.1 Pin sepsis

Grade I	Settled with improved pin care
Grade II	As above + required or received antibiotics
Grade III	As above but pin removed for sepsis
Grade IV	Sepsis persisted, despite pin removal; ring sequestrum

within the pin hole; or excessive motion between the pin and adjacent tissue.

Abscess formation

Fluid collecting around the pin drains at the surface of the soft tissue and becomes contaminated by micro-organisms. As it dries, a crust is formed around the pin/skin interface, which restricts free drainage of contaminated fluid and may subsequently lead to deep abscess formation. This argument belongs to the school of thought holding that crust removal is an essential part of pin management.

Necrotic tissue

Skin necrosis occurs with skin tension, at introduction of the pin or subsequent change in limb length or alignment.

Soft tissue necrosis occurs if the pin displaces soft tissue after being introduced through the skin. It can also occur if tissue coils up around a drill or pin not inserted through a drill sleeve.

Matthews and Hirsch[20] have reported temperature increases in bone due to the use of power drills, resulting in bone necrosis. Thermal damage can be reduced if a hand drill is used and if drilling precedes pin insertion.

It is also believed that excessive compression of the fracture, easily occurring with an external fixator, can cause bone necrosis of the pin/bone interface. This may provide an argument against pre-stressing of pin clusters.

Excessive motion

Excessive relative motion between the pin and adjacent soft tissues results in pin sepsis. In order to understand the mechanism, it is necessary to consider the inflammatory reaction and the role of chemotaxis. Phagocytic cells migrate towards micro-organisms by following a chemotactic gradient, the micro-organism itself being the source of that gradient. Environmental motion disturbs the chemotactic gradient, resulting in reduced phagocytic efficiency and sepsis (Figure 12.7).

It is likely that the low incidence of pin tract infections noted in series using the 'pins in plaster' technique is due to limited soft tissue movement.

It can be seen that, where possible, pins should be inserted through areas with minimal subcutaneous tissue, for example, the anteromedial tibial surface.

Bulky gauze, firm sponge or foam dressings between the skin and fixator should help to reduce pin/soft tissue motion.

Pin loosening within the bone has been considered the most significant factor in pin hole sepsis.[21] Chao and Pope[22] have stated that the pin/bone interface determines the stability of a frame; for this reason, it is preferable to use threaded rather than smooth pins.

Chao has shown that the stiffness of the fixator can be increased in several ways. These include increasing the number, stiffness and diameter of pins, increasing

Figure 12.8 Non-axial alignment: the frame is not parallel to the bone, which reduces axial movement.

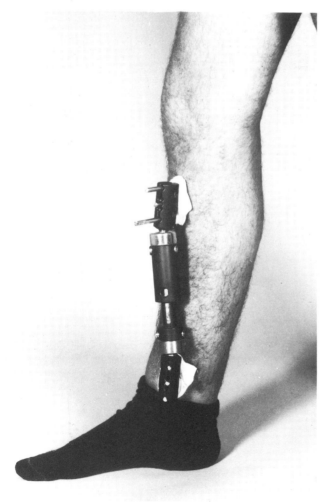

the distance between pins within the clamp, and inserting them closer to the fracture site. It is also known that aligning the fixator closer to the bone increases the rigidity of the frame.

Frame design

Improvement in frame design has been consistent in the history of external fixation, and now sophisticated frames with given degrees of rigidity are available. There is substantial lack of knowledge as to the requirements of a frame, and it is vital to consider the biology of normal fracture healing (see Chapter 4).

According to McKibbin,[23] when considering any account of fracture healing, it must be remembered that healing is a normal repair process that will occur without surgical intervention. It is vital to know the way in which treatment may alter that process. Natural healing occurs with callus formation. Direct bone union depends on accurate reduction and rigid fixation; Perren[24] has stated that direct union will not occur if there is movement at the fracture in excess of 5 to 10 μ. It is difficult to produce such slight movement at the fracture site using external fixation. Therefore, in the past many fractures were left to heal slowly; this was because the fixator provided too much rigidity to allow natural callus formation, which essentially requires movement, but insufficient rigidity for direct bone union.

The work of Vidal and of Burny perhaps epitomizes the two schools of thought. Both workers used the Hoffman components: Vidal constructed a highly rigid, double-sided quadrilateral frame; while Burny's single-sided, uniplanar device, the elastic fixator, was aimed at healing with periosteal callus.

However, although it is known that movement is required for callus formation, the questions of how much, in what direction or combination of directions, and timing, remain unanswered.

Most authors agree that shearing forces across a fracture are harmful, although Gentile[25] believes that they may be used in fracture healing.

Yamagishi and Yoshimura[26] studied 120 rabbits with experimental tibial osteotomies held with a variety of external fixators. They noted that the best healing, determined radiographically and histologically, was observed with the use of a fixator which allowed a small degree of axial movement.

Goodship and Kenwright[27] have used the Oxford Mark II, a unilateral uniplanar fixator, fitted with a device to provide controlled axial displacement, both in experiments and practice. These surgeons have reported a more rapid appearance of callus and an earlier increase of healing fracture stiffness in a group

of sheep subjected to controlled axial micromovement, compared to a control group.

De Bastiani, Aldegheri and Renzi Brivio[28] have studied 228 patients with fresh fractures treated with the Orthofix dynamic axial fixator. This allows axial movement with loading of the fracture, when the surgeon feels that the latter is sufficiently stable to permit it.

The role of axial movement seems very important. However, McKibbin[29] has reported periosteal healing with abundant callus formation, using an elastic plate which allows rotation and bending movements with little axial displacement. He warns against the belief that axial movement alone is important. McKibbin has also suggested[30] that movement may be required from the start of, not just during, the healing process.

Therefore, sufficient fundamental work on fracture healing needs to be carried out before the clinician is able to present the engineer with precise fixator requirements.

Delayed union

Delayed union frequently occurs in fractures treated with external fixators, for a variety of reasons. The most important of these has been the type of fracture. Traditionally, injuries thought to require external fixation have been high velocity, compound tibial fractures, often with gross comminutions. These have naturally had a poor prognosis.

Two other factors have already been discussed: inhibited periosteal callus formation due to the rigidity of the frame, with a lack of dynamic loading of the bone, and failure to achieve primary bone union because the frame has permitted more than 5 μ of movement. A further reason for delayed union has been the tendency of traditional external fixators to maintain a fracture gap, thus not permitting a degree of collapse which would have occurred with the limb immobilized in a cast.

More recently, attention has been drawn to the fact that an increasing number of people recognize the advantages of external fixation in treating simpler fractures than would have been considered appropriate in the past. Pringle[31] has noted delayed healing in a number of cases where the tibial fracture is without a fibular fracture, where early fibular union has developed, or with an accompanying high fibular fracture in which stability is provided by the interosseous membrane. Pringle has also suggested that delayed dynamization of the fracture by frame unlocking, using the dynamic axial fixator, is associated with delayed union, as predicted by McKibbin.

It is also recognized that a dynamic axial fixator must be fitted parallel to the bones in all planes. Non-axial alignment can lead to delayed union, perhaps as a consequence of introducing shearing forces across the fracture (Figure 12.8).

Prevention of delayed union

It is necessary to recognize that certain injuries have suffered major violence and are likely to require early bone grafting, either at the time of initial external fixation, or as soon as soft tissues permit it. Repeated bone grafting may be required.

As described above, renewed awareness of early fibular union and consideration of fibular osteotomy may be important.

By increasingly loading the healing fracture, the surgeon hopes to stimulate callus. With a rigid frame,

this is done by progressively dismantling the frame at intervals, or by sliding the fixator further away from the bone along the pins. Alternatively, some frames have a mechanism that allows free telescopic movement as required.

It has been suggested[17,32,33] that additional internal fixation, with interfragmentary lag screws, is sometimes appropriate (Figure 12.9). This clearly implies that primary bone union, at least of some part of the fracture, is sought. The difficulties of obtaining primary bone union with rigid external skeletal fixation have already been discussed. Where interfragmentary screw fixation is used in conjunction with an elastic or dynamic fixator, attempting to combine primary union and periosteal callus healing in a single long bone shaft could produce problems. Indeed, Green[34] has recently studied a series of 20 patients with diaphyseal fractures initially managed with a

Figure 12.9 Interfragmentary screw fixation of this comminuted femoral fracture is unnecessary; alignment and length are secured by the fixator.

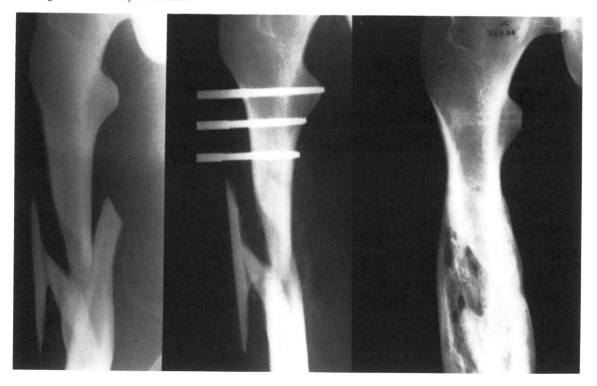

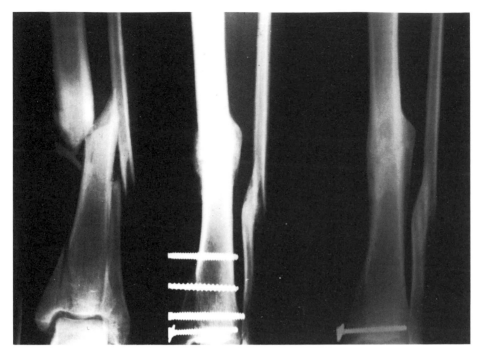

Figure 12.10 Articular surfaces should be anatomically reduced and held, as in this combined ankle and tibial fracture.

combination of external fixation and interfragmentary compression screws. About 50 per cent experienced loss of screw fixation, usually a short time after removal of the fixator. It was concluded that screw fixation may not be adequate to stabilize the fracture, unless supplemented with a bone graft.

If periosteal healing is sought, screw fixation is inappropriate and unnecessary. This does not apply where intra-articular fractures are involved. Under these circumstances it is reasonable, and perhaps even mandatory, to perform accurate joint reconstruction, with bone grafting if necessary, using internal fixation and then treating the shaft fracture as deemed appropriate (Figure 12.10).

Indications

There is disagreement among surgeons concerning the indications for external skeletal fixation. As the surgeon becomes more familiar with the application of a fixator and associated aftercare, indications may

well expand beyond the original range. However, before this happens, external fixation must show improved results compared to other methods of treatment. It should be remembered that many techniques have stood the test of time and treatment trends should not be followed without due consideration.

Compound tibial fractures

Darder and Gomar[35] have reported their experience of conservatively treated fractures, and Sarmiento[36] has demonstrated good results with early weight-bearing. The AO group[37] have also been reported on patients treated with rigid internal fixation.

However, for many surgeons, a combined Type III[38,39] soft tissue injury and comminuted tibial shaft fracture would make external fixation the obvious treatment choice (Figure 12.11): it permits wound dressings and inspections, and allows access for plastic surgery procedures if required (Figure 12.12).

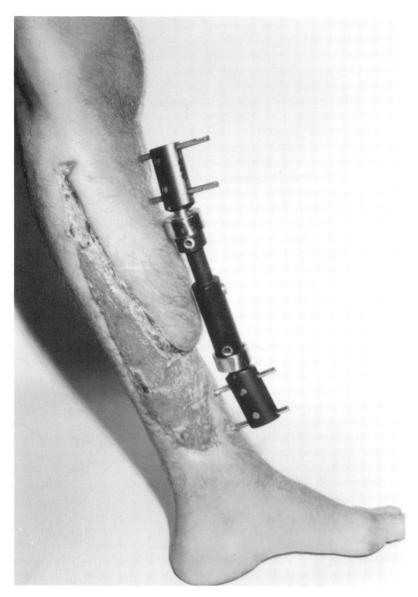

Figure 12.11 A severe Grade III open fracture treated by external fixation and skin grafting.

As stated above, such injuries often have a poor prognosis, and this may well prejudice the surgeon against external fixation for lesser injuries. Nevertheless, in many instances a fixator has helped to salvage a limb which would have otherwise required amputation. Seligson and Matheny[40] have drawn attention to the fact that a good radiographic reduction may exist beneath poor soft tissue. They have recommended a programme of aggressive treatment for such fractures, to try to reduce management complications: following initial debridement and external fixation with large half pins, the wound is treated by

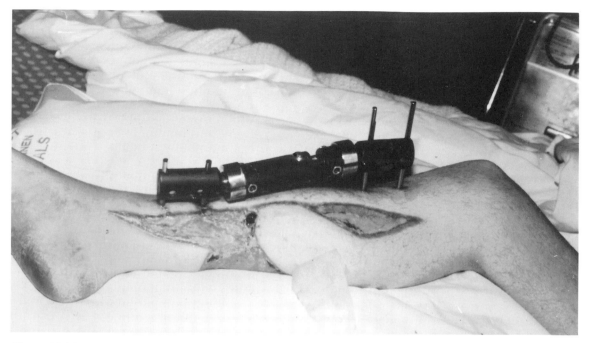

Figure 12.12 In this severe tibial fracture a rotation flap was used to cover the bone.

antibiotic beads under a plastic dressing with suction drainage. Formal plastic wound closure should be achieved by the second week, and early function and walking by the fourth week. Cancellous bone grafting is carried out by the sixth week, and after three months the frame is sequentially disassembled to increase functional loading of the bone. Following frame removal, there should be two weeks of cast protection, up to four months after injury. Seligson and Matheny point out that, due to the nature of these injuries, it is seldom possible to achieve this treatment ideal, but suggest that its application seems to reduce morbidity.

Larsson and Van der Linden[41] compared two series of patients with open tibial shaft fractures. In the first series, patients were treated conservatively with a long plaster cast, windowed, if necessary, for wound treatment, and sometimes preceded by a short period of traction. Their second series of patients with moderate or severe displacement, and Type II or III

wounds, were treated with external fixation using a modified Hoffman device. The authors had previously reported on a series of patients treated with internal fixation.[42] They noted that there was no significant difference in hospital aftercare between the conservatively treated and external fixation groups, but that internal fixation caused prolonged hospitalization. However, there was late healing and an increased rate of pseudarthrosis in the conservatively treated group, compared to the external fixation group, and they stated these differences were statistically significant. Karlstrom and Olerud[43] compared the results of 111 open tibial fractures treated with the Hoffman device with their earlier results from internal fixation: the former method saved many limbs from amputation, with an excellent or good outcome in 81 per cent of patients. The authors concluded that external fixation was their preferred method of treatment in these cases, and particularly in instances of polytrauma.

Compound femoral fractures

The advantage of external fixation in compound femoral fractures has been recognized for a long time, and was described by Crile[6] in 1918. Anderson, Judet and Hoffman all used their frames for these fractures. Fellander[44] described the use of the rigid Hoffman frame for femoral injuries, but in acute open fractures only one patient in three showed union.

Coppola and Anzel[45] reported their results from the Hoffman device in 21 cases followed up to union. In those patients, prompt mobilization was necessary but, for a variety of reasons, internal fixation was considered inappropriate. Reasons included open fractures, soft tissue injury, infection and gross comminution. Most patients had suffered polytrauma, and several had ipsilateral tibial fractures. Stabilization of the femoral fractures in these 'floating knee' cases allowed proper assessment of ligamentous damage. There was a rate of 19 per cent non-union: a great improvement over Fellander's 67 per cent.

Coppola and Anzel did not find it necessary to remove the frame prematurely for instability, pin sepsis or loss of alignment. After frame removal (average 96 days), protective bracing was used until union occurred (average 6.75 months). These surgeons felt that the frame acted as a stabilizer, and that it was important to avoid over-distraction of the fracture. Although knee motion was impaired while the fixator was in place, there was subsequent recovery. They concluded that, despite the Hoffman device being neither simple nor trouble-free, in selected cases it offered distinct advantages over other methods of treatment for acute femoral fractures.

Brug, Pennig, Gähler[46] and Hasle-Seeberg recently reported on their experience of treating over 1000 cases of polytrauma, 36 per cent of which involved femoral fractures. Since using a dynamic axial fixator instead of plates or intramedullary nails in such cases they reported a 27.3 per cent drop in mortality, owing they believe to a decreased rate in late ARDS-related death.

Closed femoral fractures

Coppola and Anzel[45] did not specify what proportion of their patients had open or closed fractures, but it is assumed that a high proportion may have been open cases.

However, De Bastiani, Aldegheri and Rensi Brivio[28] reported on 101 femoral fractures, of which 92 were closed, using a dynamic axial fixator. This clearly represents a move from the generally accepted indications for external fixation. These surgeons claim that their fixator provides a stiffness comparable to that of the Hoffman double frame device in the early stages of treatment, with simple conversion to a dynamic frame with callus enhancement, when appropriate. The fixator is left in place until union takes place, without bracing. Ninety of 92 closed femoral fractures healed in an average time of 4.4 months, and eight of nine open fractures healed in an average time of 6.5 months.

Our experience of 18 closed femoral fractures involves two refractures after removal of the fixator, and an average time to union of 18.4 weeks.[18] Advantages of this treatment include early weight-bearing, joint mobilization and no need of hospitalization, in addition to the risks of internal fixation being avoided.

Closed tibial fractures

Burny[14] has championed the role of the external fixator in closed tibial fractures, arguing that good vascularization and functional loading are essential for bone healing. He felt that, in routine fracture management, a simple frame is usually sufficient. The treatment of 1421 fractures, open as well as closed, was considered. Burny advocated the technique of a 'minimal approach' with precise reduction, without periosteal disturbance, through a 3 to 4 cm incision. Excellent results were achieved in 91.5 per cent of cases, with a mean healing time of three months for simple fractures and six months for complex fractures.

This policy of using external fixation for simple tibial fractures is echoed by the Veronese group:[28] 91 closed tibial fractures were treated to union, with a healing rate of 91 per cent in 3.6 months.

Non-union and associated infection

Vidal and colleagues[33] have recognized the importance of stability in the treatment of non-unions, with or without sepsis. They advocate initial removal of previous internal fixation, followed by radical excision of infected bone and soft tissue. Then a rigid Hoffman device is applied, the mounting pattern depending on the site: with compression in stable fractures, neutralization in unstable fractures, and with distraction where bone loss has occurred. Following this initial stage, the authors describe an intermediate phase during which granulation develops on the pseudarthrosis site. They use continuous irrigation to help stimulate the formation of granulated tissue. This phase is complete when

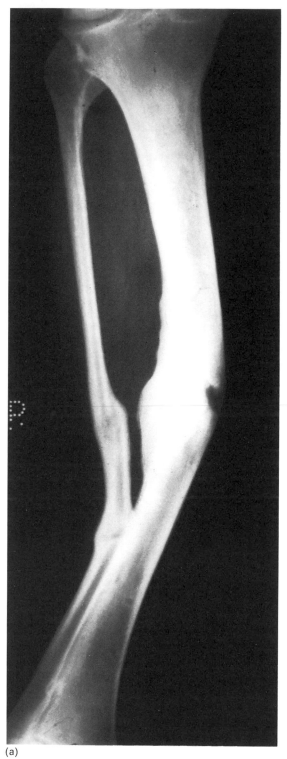
(a)

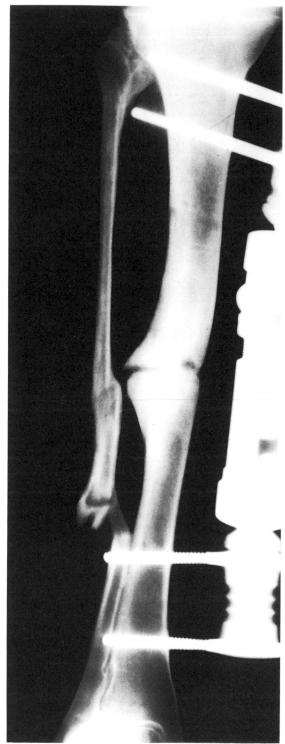
(b)

Figure 12.13 *a* and *b* An external fixation frame used to correct angular malalignment following conservative management.

infection is controlled and skin cover has occurred. The final phase, or secondary treatment, involves osseous consolidation, achieved in a number of ways: for example, in a stable lesion, such as a hypertrophic non-union, compression is applied with or without initial osteomuscular decortication. The compression is checked every two weeks.

For unstable lesions, early inter-tibiofibular grafting is recommended. The Papineau technique is indicated in partial loss of bone. For substantial bone loss, a cross-leg flap follows preliminary inter-tibio-fibular grafting. Recently, microsurgical techniques have been developed, such as vascularized fibula transplantation and the highly successful composite inguino-iliac flap, in combination with external fixation.

Agostini and Leso[47] have recently reported the results from using the dynamic axial fixator in 85 cases of pseudarthrosis. Of those, 44 involved the tibia, 24 the femur, and the remainder involved the humerus and radius; there was also a case of ulnar pseudarthrosis. Seventy-two cases were aseptic. Hypertrophic cases were treated with the frame in compression, with or without 'muscular bone decortication', and partial excision of the fibula where necessary. There was a healing rate of 94 per cent in aseptic and 77 per cent in septic cases, with a mean healing time of 157 days. Undoubtedly, many will agree that the external fixator is invaluable in the management of such cases.

Similarly, in cases of malunion, the external fixator can be a valuable tool for stabilizing the limb after correction of malalignment (Figure 12.13).

Pelvis

Seligson[48] gave an account of the history of external fixation in pelvic injuries, and pointed out that the lack of their classification into different therapeutic groups has hampered progress significantly. The classification by Tile and Pennal[49] has been received as a helpful advance.

In anteroposterior compression injuries, the pelvis opens with a pubic diastasis. This can be treated with an anterior frame, such as the dynamic axial fixator, or a simple Hoffman device (Figure 12.14).

In lateral compression injuries, there is either a fracture near the sacroiliac joint, or the posterior sacroiliac ligaments are torn. For these Seligson advocates the use of the compressive trapezoidal frame described by Slatis and Karaharju,[50] with Hoffman components.

Injuries involving a vertical shear are more complex. Disruption of the anterior and posterior ligaments, or of the bony pelvis, allows upward displacement of the injured segment. Longitudinal traction is required to reduce the deformity; the position is held with a combination of external fixation anteriorly and internal fixation posteriorly, or a very stable, double anteroposterior frame.

External fixation in upper limb injuries

The upper limb is generally well-treated by other methods, but sometimes external fixation may be considered.

Vidal and Nakach[51] recently suggested that external fixation would be appropriate in the following instances: severe open fractures, some cases of arthrodesis of the shoulder or elbow, and unstable wrist injuries (ligamentotaxis: Figure 12.15).

Cooney[52] described the experience of the Mayo Clinic between 1975 and 1984, regarding these injuries: of 40 cases, nine were fractures of the humerus, nine were fractures of one of the forearm bones, and 26 were fractures of both forearm bones. The external fixator was applied for an average of nine weeks, followed by casting or delayed open reduction and internal fixation. Cooney's treatment goals included limb salvage, fracture union, improved function and patient satisfaction. A satisfactory result was obtained in 72 per cent of cases, although there was a delayed union rate of 34 per cent which required bone grafting. There were two amputations in failed limb salvage due to secondary sepsis. External fixation was reserved for unstable injuries with significant soft tissue or neurovascular injury requiring skeletal stability and wound access to facilitate limb salvage.

By contrast, Lavini and Mosconi[53] reported a series of 81 upper limb fractures during the period 1980–85, 56 of which were fractures of the humerus; the majority involved closed treatment, with an average healing time of 3.4 months. The authors' justification for this policy, as opposed to other methods, was the rapid return of function.

External fixation in articular fractures

Vidal and colleagues[54] have pointed out that it is not always possible to reconstruct intra-articular fractures composed of many small pieces, as these prohibit compression. In these epiphyseal injuries, the force producing the fracture is usually compressive, leaving the capsule and ligaments intact. After pins are inserted above and below the injured joint, they are distracted, thus realigning the fracture fragments

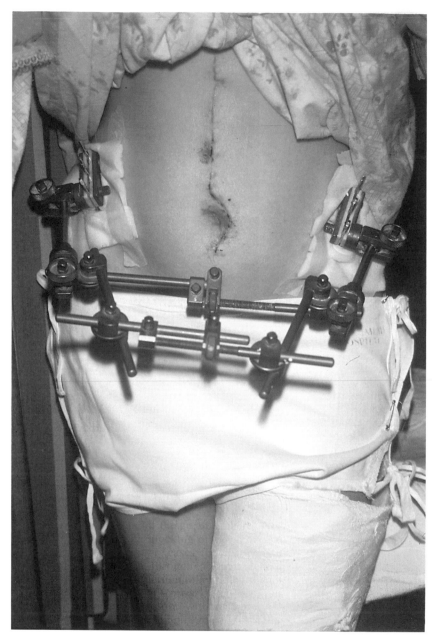

Figure 12.14 A Hoffman pelvic A frame.

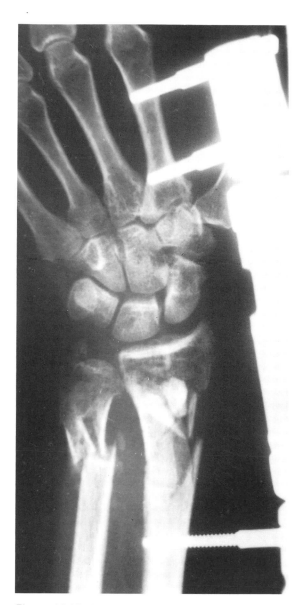

Figure 12.15 The principle of ligamentotaxis is used to hold a good correction of a severe distal radial fracture.

Mini-fixator

A variety of mini-fixators are available for injuries of digits and metacarpals. Their use is not yet widespread, although they were mentioned in six papers read at a conference entitled Recent Advances in External Fixation, in Riva del Garda, Italy, in September 1986.

Discussion focused on stability and preservation of hand mobility: the role of the fixator in digital and metacarpal fractures, stabilization during arthrodesis for post-traumatic oesteoarthritis of small joints, and lengthening of digits and metacarpals.

Fractures in children

Ombredanne[55] first recommended external fixation in children, emphasizing that only a short period of fixation is required, there is a reduced risk of infection, and additional surgery is unnecessary for implant removal.

O'Connor[56] holds that indications for external (or internal) fixation in children must be few, but Stanwyck and Seligson,[57] reporting on ten cases, suggest that this technique is perhaps underused in the management of complex paediatric fractures, particularly in cases of polytrauma.

Arthrodesis

Arthrodesis is still performed as a primary procedure for some orthopaedic conditions and post-traumatic osteoarthritis, although it is mainly used as a salvage procedure following failed joint replacement. Green[17] has reviewed the subject, drawing attention to the causes of unsuccessful arthrodesis and to Charnley's outline of compression arthrodesis.[58] Although the aim is to produce two congruous cancellous surfaces, Charnley pointed out that where this ideal is not achieved, rigid contact at one point will be followed by union across the beachhead (providing there is no shearing motion), with subsequent union across the cancellous surfaces.

Lance, Paval, Fries, Larsen and Patterson[59] noted that, over a 20-year period, arthrodesis of the ankle, using external fixation, resulted in a higher union rate (94 per cent) compared to other techniques. Ratliff[60] also noted that Charnley's technique gave satisfactory results. However, in cases of post-traumatic arthritis of the hip, knee and elbow without a history of joint sepsis, it may be that internal fixation is preferable to external fixation.

and preserving the joint space. These surgeons have used this method in the hip, knee, ankle and other joints, and suggest that it works best in the wrist, particularly if joint movement is possible.

Spine

Certain types of spinal fracture may be amenable to external fixation. Magerl[61] outlined its advantages over conventional internal fixation in spinal fractures, suggesting that only three, instead of five, vertebrae need to be immobilized, with no additional external support (as opposed to internal fixation which requires additional bracing). Magerl used four Schanz screws, inserted through the pedicles into the vertebral bodies under radiographic control, and connected by an adjustable external frame (Figure 12.16). He has reported the results from 77 patients, out of approximately 100 treated since 1977. Of these, 62 were fracture cases, 32 of them having significant neurological complications. Walking was possible after six days on average, and hospitalization ceased

at 26 days. The fixator was removed at 17 weeks on average. Excellent results were noted in 33 patients, good in 15, fair in 12, and poor in two patients.

Complications included loss of correction in four cases and pin loosening in three cases; seroma, superficial wound infection and pin tract infection each occurred in one case.

Olerud, Sjostrom, Hamberg and Karlstrom[62] have also described the use of external fixation in the spine, particularly as a diagnostic and therapeutic aid in the management of chronic low back pain. Out of 62 patients treated, four who had undergone previous spinal surgery were noted to have leakage of cerebrospinal fluid after removal of the fixator. This leakage settled without untoward effect, but it is likely to deter most surgeons from using external skeletal fixation as a routine measure for spinal fractures.

Figure 12.16 *a* The Dick spinal fixator used to hold reduction of an anterior spinal osteotomy and fusion for congenital kyphosis; *b* spinal transpedicular Schanz screws are attached to the external fixator frame.

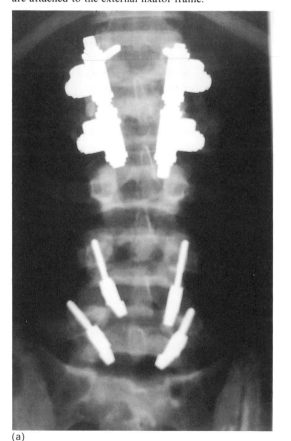

(a)

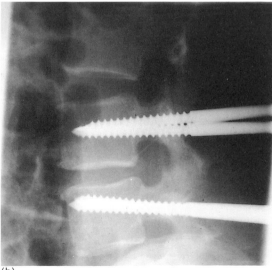

(b)

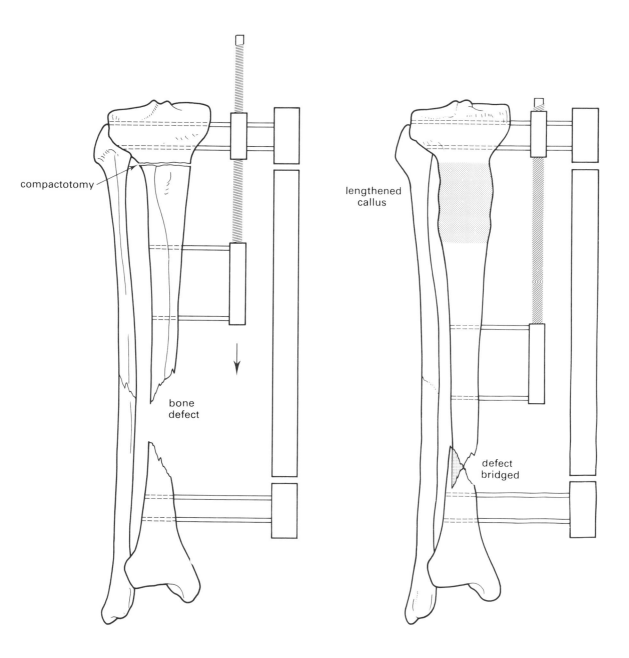

compactotomy

bone
defect

lengthened
callus

defect
bridged

Figure 12.17 The method pioneered by Ilisarov to close
a segmental defect in the lower tibia; a proximal
osteotomy is created and the callus distracted, moving the
central fragment down to close the defect. Although
Ilisarov pioneered this technique using his ring fixator, for
reasons of clarity a monolateral is used schematically in
the illustration.

Facial fractures

Such fractures are generally treated by maxillofacial surgeons. The subject is covered in depth by Rowe and Williams.[63]

Corrective osteotomies for malunion

External fixation may be used for axial correction in orthopaedic conditions, such as medial compartment osteoarthrosis of the knee,[64,65] but also in correcting fracture malunion.[66]

This can be achieved by traditional surgery and also the 'hemicallotasi' method, originally described by the Verona group and recently advocated by Turi, Tomasi, Arnotti and Cassini:[63] this technique involves a hemicorticotomy, without the medullary cavity being traversed if possible, and after an appropriate period of partial weight-bearing (in the region of 14 days), radiographic evidence of early callus is sought. This callus is subsequently distracted, creating an opening wedge of new bone and thus correcting the malalignment.

The future

New concepts in pin design have introduced different threads for various locations, maximal size of pins that does not compromise the compressibility factor of bone, tapering pins allowing some possibility of further introduction, and tightening of pins in the early stages of loosening.

Undoubtedly, new material will be developed for connecting bodies. These may be of reduced torsional stiffness, such as carbon fibre, to encourage the production of periosteal callus.

Future fixators will monitor fracture healing.[67] A number of methods may be suitable, such as strain gauging or monitoring of acoustic emission. Possibly digital readout would enable the suitably informed patient to recognize abnormal patterns of fracture healing, resulting in the early diagnosis of delayed or non-union. A microprocessor may instruct the fixator when weight-bearing is appropriate. Delayed union may be treated with the use of electrical stimulation via the external fixation pins.

Improvements of surgical techniques would include education of the staff involved in applying and caring for external fixators, including nurses responsible for postoperative care.

At present, slit or cruciate skin incisions are performed, which do not evenly accommodate a circular pin. A circular skin hole caused, for example, by a suction apparatus in conjunction with a guillotine knife may reduce skin tension problems.

New surgical techniques will continue to be developed. Gallinaro, Biasibetti and Demangos[68] recently discussed their experience of increasing bone stock in pseudarthrosis with bone loss: following initial compression of the pseudarthrosis to promote fracture union, the healing non-union was distracted to restore length.

Gallinaro, Rossi, Dettoni and Agnese[69] described an even more exciting technique, using the Ilisarov fixator in severe open tibial fractures with bone and skin loss. Having applied a fixator to the injured limb, they carried out a 'closed compactotomy', that is, corticotomy, in the segment of bone above the injury. The bone was then distracted at the corticotomy site, with progressive filling of the gap; the bone segment and soft tissue would descend, replacing the lost area of bone and soft tissue (Figure 12.17).

However, improvements in the design and structure of pins, pin grippers and connecting bodies depend on the surgeon's ability to describe all requirements to the design engineer. This knowledge must depend on an improved understanding of the process of fracture repair and the ways in which it can be influenced, for example by movement, as indicated earlier.

Such exciting proposals have been summarized by De Bastiani in his statement that, 'The applications of external fixation are limited only by the fantasies of the surgical mind' (G De Bastiani, personal communication, 1986).

References

Chapter 1

1 Mast G, AO Instructional course lecture, Davos, 1982.
2 Müller ME, Allgower M, Schneider R, et al, *Manual of internal fixation, techniques recommended by the AO group*, 2nd edition (Springer: Berlin, Heidelberg, New York, 1977).
3 Van Gorder GW, Surgical approaches in supracondylar 'T' fractures of the distal humerus requiring open reduction, *J Bone Joint Surg* (1940) **22**: 278–92.

Chapter 2

1 Nicaise E, *La grande chirurgie de Guy de Chauliac* (Paris, 1890).
2 Mee A, *The King's England: Nottinghamshire* (Hodder and Stoughton: London, 1938).
3 Paré A, *The works of Ambroise Paré* (translated and published by T Johnson: London, 1691).
4 Godlee R, *Lord Lister* (Macmillan: London, 1917).
5 Lister J, On a new method of treating compound fractures, abscesses etc, *Lancet* (1867) **i**: 326.
6 Friedrich PL, Die aseptisches Versurgung frischer Wunden, *Arch Klin Chir* (1898) **57**: 300–309.
7 Watson F, *The life of Sir Robert Jones* (Hodder and Stoughton: London, 1934).
8 Trueta J, Closed treatment of war fractures, *Lancet* (1939) **i**: 1452–5.
9 Winnett Orr H, Treatment of acute osteomyelitis by drainage and rest, *J Bone Joint Surg* (1927) **9**: 733–9.
10 Heaton LD, Hughes CW, Rosegay H et al, Military surgical practices of the United States Army in Vietnam, *Curr Prob Surg* (1966) 1–59.
11 Gustilo RB, Anderson JT, Prevention of infection in the treatment of one thousand and twenty-five open fractures of long bones, *J Bone Joint Surg* (1976) **58A**: 453–8.
12 Patzakis MJ, Ivler D, Antibiotic and bacteriologic considerations in open fractures, *Southern Med J* (1977) **70**: 46–8.
13 Cooney WP, Fitzgerald RH, Dobyns JH et al, Quantitative wound cultures in upper extremity trauma, *J Trauma* (1982) **22**: 112–17.
14 Marshall KA, Ederton MT, Rodeheaver GT et al, Quantitative microbiology: its application to hand injuries, *Am J Surg* (1976) **131**: 730–3.
15 Robson MC, Duke WF, Krizek TJ, Rapid bacterial screening in the treatment of civilian wounds, *J Surg Res* (1973) **14**: 426–30.
16 Edlich RF, Rogers W, Kaspar G et al, Studies in the management of the contaminated wound: 1) Optimal time for closure of contaminated wounds; 2) Comparison of resistance to infection of open and closed wounds during healing, *Am J Surg* (1969) **117**: 583–91.
17 Miles AA, Miles E, Burke JF, The value and duration of defence reactions of the skin to the primary lodgement of bacteria, *Brit J Exp Path* (1957) **38**: 79–96.
18 Burke JF, The effective period of preventative antibiotic action in experimental incisions and dermal lesions, *Surgery* (1961) **50**: 161–8.
19 Polk, HC, Miles AA, The decisive period in the primary infection of muscle by *Escherichia coli*, *Br J Exp Path* (1973) **54**: 99–109.
20 Patzakis MJ, Management of open fractures, *American Academy of Orthopaedic Surgeons, Instructional Course Lectures* (1982) **31**: 62–4.
21 Howard RJ, Simmons RL, Acquired immunologic deficiencies after trauma and surgical procedures, *Surg Gynecol Obstet* (1974) **139**: 771–82.
22 Mader JT, Cierny G, The principles of the use of preventative antibiotics, *Clin Orthop* (1984) **190**: 75–82.
23 Gustilo RB, Management of open fractures and complications, *American Academy of Orthopaedic Surgeons, Instructional Course Lectures* (1982) **31**: 64–75.
24 Gustilo RB, Mendoza RM, Williams DN, Problems in the management of Type III (severe) open fractures: a new classification of Type III open fractures, *J Trauma* (1984) **24**: 742–6.
25 Patzakis MJ, Harvey JP, Ivler D, The role of antibiotics in the management of open fractures, *J Bone Joint Surg* (1974) **56A**: 532–41.
26 Tscherne H, Oestern HJ, Sturm J, Osteosynthesis of major fractures in polytrauma, *World J Surg* (1983) **7**: 80–7.
27 Worlock PH, Slack RCB, Harvey L et al, The prevention of infection in experimental open fractures: the effect of antibiotics, *J Bone Joint Surg (Am)* (1988) **70A**: 1341–7.
28 Müller ME, Allgower M, Schneider R et al, *Manual of internal fixation*, 2nd edition (Springer: Berlin, Heidelberg, New York, 1979).
29 Rittmann WW, Schibli M, Matter P et al, Open fractures: long term results in 200 consecutive cases, *Clin Orthop* (1979) **138**: 132–40.
30 Bergmann BR, Antibiotic prophylaxis in open and closed fractures: a controlled clinical trial, *Acta Orthop Scand* (1982) **53**: 57–62.
31 Brown PW, The prevention of infection in open wounds, *Clin Orthop* (1973) **96**: 42–50.
32 Epps CH, Adams JP, Wound management in open fractures, *Am Surg* (1961) **27**: 766–9.
33 Allgower M, Border JR, Management of fractures in the multiple trauma patient, *World J Surg* (1983) **7**: 88–95.
34 Chapman MW, Role of bone stability in open fractures, *American Academy of Orthopaedic Surgeons, Instructional Course Lectures* (1982) **31**: 75–87.
35 Burri C, *Post-traumatic osteomyelitis* (Hans Huber: Berne, 1975).

36 Weber BG, Cech O, *Pseudarthrosis* (Hans Huber: Berne, 1976).

37 Rittmann WW, Perren SM, *Cortical bone healing after internal fixation and infection* (Springer: Berlin, Heidelberg, New York, 1974).

38 Friedrich B, Klaue P, Mechanical stability and post-traumatic osteitis: an experimental evaluation of the relation between infection of bone and internal fixation, *Injury* (1977) **9**: 23–9.

39 Worlock PH, The prevention of infection in open fractures. An experimental study of the effects of fracture stability and of antibiotic therapy, DM thesis, University of Nottingham, 1987.

40 Selye H, *The stress of life* (McGraw-Hill: New York, 1956).

41 Khan DS, Pritzker KPH, The pathophysiology of bone infection, *Clin Orthop* (1973) **96**: 12–19.

42 Rhinelander FW, Phillips RS, Steel WM et al, Micro-angiography in bone healing. III) Osteotomies with internal fixation, *J Bone Joint Surg* (1967) **49A**: 1006–1007.

43 Ganz R, Brennwald J, Hunter W et al, The recovery of medullary circulation after osteotomy and internal fixation, *Europ Surg Res* (1970) **2**: 106.

44 Sarmiento A, Latta LL, *Closed functional treatment of fractures* (Springer: Berlin, Heidelberg, New York, 1981).

45 Green SA, Complications of external skeletal fixation, *Clin Orthop* (1983) **180**: 109–16.

46 Velazco A, Fleming LL, Open fractures of the tibia treated by the Hoffman external fixator, *Clin Orthop* (1983) **180**: 125–32.

47 Clifford RP, Lyons TJ, Webb JK, Complications of external fixation of compound tibial fractures, *Injury* (1987) **18**: 174–6.

48 Wade PA, Campbell RD, Open versus closed methods in treating fractures of the leg, *Am J Surg* (1958) **95**: 599–616.

49 Claffey T, Open fractures of the tibia, *J Bone Joint Surg* (1960) **42B**: 407.

50 Gallinaro P, Crova M, Denicolai F, Complications in 64 open fractures of the tibia, *Injury* (1973) **5**: 157–60.

51 Chapman MW, Mahoney M, The role of early internal fixation in the management of open fractures, *Clin Orthop* (1979) **138**: 120–31.

52 Clifford RP, Webb JK, Beauchamp CG et al, Plate fixation of open fractures of the tibia, *J Bone Joint Surg (Br)* (1988) **70B**: 644–8.

53 Moed BR, Kellam JF, Foster RJ et al, Immediate internal fixation of open fractures of the diaphysis of the forearm, *J Bone Joint Surg* (1986) **68A**: 1008–17.

54 Bell MJ, Beauchamp CG, Kellam JF et al, The results of plating humeral shaft fractures in patients with multiple injuries, *J Bone Joint Surg* (1985) **67B**: 293–6.

55 La Duca JN, Bone LL, Seibel RW et al, Primary open reduction and internal fixation of open fractures, *J Trauma* (1980) **20**: 580–6.

56 Hicks JH, The relationship between metal and infection, *Proc Roy Soc Med* (1957) **50**: 842–4.

57 Zimmerli W, Waldvogel FA, Vaudaux P et al, Pathogenesis of foreign body infection: description and characteristics of an animal model, *J Infect Dis* (1982) **146**: 487–97.

58 Christensen GD, Simpson WA, Bisno AL et al, Experimental foreign body infections in mice challenged with slime-producing *Staphylococcus epidermis*, *Infect Immun* (1983) **40**: 407–10.

59 Southwood RT, Rice JL, McDonald PJ et al, Infection in experimental hip arthroplasties, *J Bone Joint Surg* (1985) **67B**: 229–31.

60 Schatzker J, Open intramedullary nailing of the femur, *Orthop Clin North Am* (1980) **11**: 623–31.

61 Weller S, Kuner E, Schweikert CH, Medullary nailing according to Swiss Study Group principles, *Clin Orthop* (1979) **138**: 45–55.

62 Winquist RA, Hansen ST, Clawson DK, Closed intramedullary nailing of femoral fractures, *J Bone Joint Surg* (1984) **66A**: 529–39.

63 Cleveland, M, Grove JA, Delayed primary closure of wounds with compound fractures, *J Bone Joint Surg* (1945) **27**: 452–6.

Chapter 3

1 Gustilo RB, Anderson JT, Prevention of infection in the treatment of one thousand and twenty-five open fractures of long bones, *J Bone Joint Surg* (1976) **58A**: 453–8.

2 Brown RF, The management of traumatic tissue loss in the lower limb, especially when complicated by skeletal injury, *Br J Plast Surg* (1965) **18**: 26–50.

3 Olerud S, Karlstrom G, Danckwardt-Lilliestrom G, Treatment of open fractures of the tibia and ankle, *Clin Orthop* (1978) **136**: 212–24.

4 Clifford RP, Webb JK, Beauchamp CG et al, Plate fixation of open fractures of the tibia, *J Bone Joint Surg* (1988): **70B**: 644–8.

5 Godina M, Early microsurgical reconstruction of complex trauma of the extremities, *Plast Reconstr Surg* (1986) **78:3**: 285–92.

6 Cierny G, Byrd HS, Jones RE, Primary versus delayed soft tissue coverage for severe open tibial fractures, *Clin Orthop* (1983) **178**: 54–63.

7 James MI, McGrouther DA, Delayed exposed skin grafting: a 10 year experience of the technique, *Br J Plast Surg* (1985) **38**: 124–8.

8 Davison PM, Batchelor AG, Lewis-Smith PA, The properties and uses of non-expanded machine-meshed skin grafts, *Br J Plast Surg* (1986) **39**: 462–8.

9 Jackson IT, Flaps: Design and management, in: *Recent Advances in Plastic Surgery 1*, Ed Calman J (Churchill Livingstone: Edinburgh, London, New York, 1976).

10 Stranc MF, Labandter H, Roy A, A review of 196 tubed pedicles, *Br J Plast Surg* (1975) **28**: 54–8.

11 Cannon B, Lischer CE, Davis WB et al, The use of open jump flaps in lower extremity repairs, *Plast Reconstr Surg* (1947) **2**: 336–41.

12 Dawson RLG, Complications of the cross-leg flap operation, *Proc Roy Soc Med* (1972) **65**: 626–9.

13 McGregor IA, Morgan G, Axial and random pattern flaps, *Br J Plast Surg* (1973) **26**: 202–13.

14 Haertsch PA, The blood supply to the skin of the leg: a postmortem investigation, *Br J Plast Surg* (1981) **34**: 470–7.

15 Cormack GC, Lamberty BGH, A classification of

fasciocutaneous flaps according to their patterns of vascularisation, *Br J Plast Surg* (1984) **37**: 80–87.

16   Tolhurst DE, Haeseker B, Zeeman RJ, The development of the fasciocutaneous flap and its clinical applications, *Plast Reconstr Surg* (1983) **71:5**: 597–605.

17   Aclamd RD, Schusterman M, Godina M et al, The saphenous neurovascular free flap, *Plast Reconstr Surg* (1981) **67:6**: 763–74.

18   Ger R, 'The management of pretibial skin loss', *Surgery* (1968) **63**: 757–63.

19   Pers M, Medgyesi S, Pedicle muscle flaps and their applications in the surgery of repair, *Br J Plast Surg* (1973) **26**: 313–21.

20   Mathes SJ, McCraw JB, Vasconez LO, Muscle transposition flaps for coverage of lower extremity defects, *Surg Clin N Am* (1974) **54:6**: 1337–54.

21   Dowden V, McCraw JB, Myocutaneous flaps, in: *Recent Advances in Plastic Surgery 2*, Ed Jackson IT (Churchill Livingstone: Edinburgh, London, New York, 1981).

22   Nahai F, Mathes SJ, Musculocutaneous flap or muscle flap and skin graft? *Ann Plast Surg* (1984) **12:2**: 199–203.

23   McCraw JB, Selection of alternative local flaps in the leg and foot, *Clin Plast Surg* (1979) **6:2**: 227–46.

24   Ponten B, The fasciocutaneous flap: its use in soft tissue defects of the lower leg, *Br J Plast Surg* (1981) **34**: 215–20.

25   Barclay TL, Cardoso E, Sharpe DT, et al, Repair of lower leg injuries with fasciocutaneous flaps, *Br J Plast Surg* (1982) **35**: 127–32.

26   Thatte RL, Yelikar AD, Chhajlami P et al, Successful detachment of cross-leg fasciocutaneous flaps on the tenth day: a report of 10 cases, *Br J Plast Surg* (1986) **39**: 491–7.

27   Krizek TJ, Tami T, Desprez JD et al, Experimental transplantation of composite grafts by microsurgical vascular anastomosis, *Plast Reconstr Surg* (1965) **36**: 538–46.

28   Komatso S, Tamai S, Successful replantation of a completely cut-off thumb, *Plast Reconstr Surg* (1968) **42**: 374–7.

29   Cobbett J, Free digit transfer: a report of a case of transfer of a great toe to replace an amputated thumb, *J Bone Joint Surg* (1969) **51B**: 677–9.

30   Daniel RG, Taylor GI, Distant transfer of an island flap by microvascular anastomosis, *Plast Reconstr Surg* (1973) **52:2**: 111–17.

31   Taylor GI, Miller GDH, Ham FJ, The free vascularised bone graft, *Plast Reconstr Surg* (1975) **55:5**: 533–44.

32   Harii K, Ohmoni K, Torii S, Free gracilis muscle transplantation with microneurovascular anastomosis for the treatment of facial paralysis, *Plast Reconstr Surg* (1976) **57**: 133–43.

33   Taylor GI, Ham FJ, The free vascularised nerve graft, *Plast Reconstr Surg* (1976) **57**: 413–26.

34   Buncke H, Furnas D, Gordon L et al, Free osteocutaneous flap from a rib to the tibia, *Plast Reconstr Surg* (1977) **59**: 799–805.

35   Taylor GI, Watson N, One stage repair of compound leg defects with free revascularised flaps of groin skin and iliac bone, *Plast Reconstr Surg* (1978) **61**: 494–506.

36   Godina M, Preferential use of end-to-side anastomosis in free flap transfer, *Plast Reconstr Surg* (1979) **64**: 673–82.

37   Hu Q, Jaang Q, Su G et al, Free vascularised bone graft, *Chin Med J* (1980) **93**: 753–7.

38   Tamai et al, Vascularised fibular transplantation: a report of eight cases in the treatment of traumatic bony defects of pseudo-arthrosis of long bones, *Int J Microsurg* (1980) **2**: 205–12.

39   Chen ZW, Yang DY, Chang DS, *Microsurgery* (Springer: Berlin, Heidelberg, New York, 1982).

40   McGregor IA, Jackson IT, The groin flap, *Br J Plast Surg* (1972) **22**: 3–16.

41   Bakamjian VY, A two-staged method for pharynoesophageal construction with a primary pectoral skin flap, *Plast Reconstr Surg* (1965) **36**: 173–84.

42   Bailey BN, Godfrey AM, Latissimus dorsi muscle free flaps, *Br J Plast Surg* (1982) **35**: 47–52.

43   Taylor GI, Composite tissue transfer to the lower limb, in *Recent Advances in Plastic Surgery 3*, Eds Jackson IT and Sommerland BC (Churchill Livingstone: Edinburgh, London, New York, 1985).

44   Taylor GI, Corlett R, Boyd JB, The extended deep inferior epigastric flap; a clinical technique, *Plast Reconstr Surg* (1983) **72:6**: 751–64.

45   Taylor GI, Corlett RJ, Boyd JB, The versatile deep inferior epigastric (inferior rectus abdominis) flap, *Br J Plast Surg* (1984) **37**: 330–50.

46   Zook, EG, Russel RC, Asaadi M, A comparative study of free and pedicle flaps for lower extremity wounds, *Ann Plast Surg* (1986) **17**: 21–33.

47   Taylor GI, Townsend P, Corlett R, Superiority of the deep circumflex iliac vessels as the supply for free groin flaps, *Plast Reconstr Surg* (1979) **64:6**: 745–59.

48   Donski PK, Buchler V, Ganz R, Combined osteocutaneous microvascular flap procedure for extensive bone and soft tissue defects in the tibia, *Ann Plast Surg* (1986) **16:5**: 386–98.

49   Wei, FC, Chen HC, Chuang CC et al, Fibular osteoseptocutaneous flap; anatomic study and clinical application, *Plast Reconstr Surg* (1986) **78:2**: 191–9.

50   Cormack GC, Duncan MJ, Lamberty BGH, The blood supply of the bone component of the compound osteocutaneous radial artery forearm flap—an anatomical study, *Br J Plast Surg* (1986) **39**: 173–5.

Chapter 4

1   Tonna EK, Cronkite EP, Use of tritiated thymidine for the study of the origin of osteoclast, *Nature* (1961) **190**: 459.

2   Schenk R, Willeneger H, Morphological findings in primary fracture healing, *Symposia Biologica Molecula* (1967) **8**: 75–86.

3   McKibbin B, The biology of fracture healing in long bones, *J Bone Joint Surg* (1978) **60B**: 150–62.

4   Sevitt S, *Bone repair and healing in man* (Churchill Livingstone, Edinburgh, 1981).

5   Danis R, *Théorie et pratique de l'ostéosynthèse* (Masson, Paris, 1959) 20.

6   Perren SM, Physical and biological aspects of fracture healing with special reference to internal fixation, *Clin Orthop* (1979) **138**: 175–96.

7   Charnley J, *The Closed Treatment of Common Fractures* (Churchill Livingstone, Edinburgh and London, 1972).

Chapter 5

1   Ollier L, *Traite experimental et clinique de la regeneration des os et de la production artificielle du tissue osseux* Vols I and II (Masson, Paris, 1867).
2   MacEwen W, Observations concerning transplantation of bone. Illustrated by a case of inter-human osseus transplantation, whereby over two-thirds of the shaft of a humerus are restored, *Proc R Soc Lond (Biol)* (1881) **32**: 232–47.
3   Hey Groves EW, *On modern methods of treating fractures*, 2nd edition (John Wright and Sons, Bristol, 1921).
4   Barth A, Uber histologische Befunde nach Knochenimplantation, *Arch Klin Chir* (1893) **46**: 409–17.
5   Axhausen G, Die histologischen und klinischen Gesetze der freien Osteoplastik auf Grund von Thierversuch, *Arch Klin Chir* (1908) **88**: 23–145.
6   Phemister DB, Splint grafts in the treatment of delayed and non-union of fractures, *Surg Gynecol Obstet* (1931) **52**: 376–81.
7   Gray JC, Elves MW, Donor cells' contribution to osteogenisis in experimental cancellous bone grafts, *Clin Orthop* (1982) **163**: 261–71.
8   Mowlem R, Bone and cartilage transplants, their use and behaviour, *Br J Surg* (1941) **29**: 182–93.
9   Mowlem R, Cancellous chip bone grafts. Report on 75 cases, *Lancet* (1944) **ii**: 746–8.
10   Nade S, Clinical implications of cell function in osteogenisis. A reappraisal of bone-graft surgery, *Ann R Coll Surg Engl* (1979) **6**: 189–94.
11   Burwell RG, A study of homologous cancellous bone combined with autologous red marrow after transplantation to a muscular site, *J Anat* (1961) **95**: 613.
12   Albrektsson T, In vivo studies of bone grafts. The possibility of vascular anastomosea in healing bone, *Acta Orthop Scand* (1980) **51**: 9–17.
13   Cleveland M, Winant EM, Treatment of non-union in compound fractures with infection, *J Bone Joint Surg Br* (1952) **34A**: 554–63.
14   Papineau LJ, Alfagme A, Dalcourt JP et al, Osteomyelite chronique: excision et greffe de spongieux à l'air libre, *Int Orthop* (1979) **3**: 165–76.
15   Clement DA, Szypryt EP, An experimental study in the rabbit of the role of cortico-cancellous bone graft used to augment plate fixation of a contaminated osteotomy *J Bone Joint Surg* (1987) **69B**: 496.
16   Chacha PB, Ahmed M, Daruwalla JS, Vascular pedicle graft of the ipsilateral fibula for non-union of the tibia with a large defect, *J Bone Joint Surg* (1981) **63B**: 244–53.
17   Baksi DP, Treatment of post-traumatic avascular necrosis of the femoral head by multiple drilling and muscle-pedicle bone grafting, *J Bone Joint Surg* (1983) **65B**: 268–73.
18   Leung PC, Chow YYN, Reconstruction of proximal femoral defects with a vascular-pedicled graft, *J Bone Joint Surg* (1984) **66B**: 32–7.
19   Pho RWH, Levack B, Satku K et al, Free vascularised fibula graft in the treatment of congenital pseudarthrosis of the tibia, *J Bone Joint Surg* (1985) **67B**: 64–70.
20   Taylor GI, Watson R, One-stage repair of compound leg defects with free, vascularized flaps of groin skin and iliac bone, *Plast Reconstr Surg* (1978) **61**: 494–506.
21   Friedlaender GE, Current concepts review bone-banking, *J Bone Joint Surg* (1982) **64A**: 307–11.
22   Tomford WW, Doppelt SH, Mankin HJ, 1983 bone bank procedures, *Clin Orthop* (1983) **174**: 15–21.
23   Burwell RG, The function of bone marrow in the incorporation of bone graft, *Clin Orthop* (1986) **200**: 125–41.
24   Burwell RG, Studies in the transplantation of bone VIII. Treated composite homograft-autografts of cancellous bone: an analysis of inductive mechanisms in the bone transplant, *J Bone Joint Surg* (1966) **48B**: 532–66.
25   Salama MB, Xenograft bone grafting in humans, *Clin Orthop* (1983) **174**: 113–21.
26   Urist MR, Mikulski A, Boyd SD, A chemosteralised antigen-extracted autodigested alloimplant for bone banks, *Arch Surg* (1975) **110**: 416–28.
27   Burwell RG, The fate of bone grafts, *Recent advances in orthopaedics*, Ed Apley AG (J and A Churchill: London, 1969) 115–207.
28   Huggins CB, The function of bone under the influence of epithelium of the urinary tract, *Arch Surg* (1931) **22**: 377–408.
29   Claes L, Burri C, Gerngross H et al, Bone healing stimulated by plasma factor XIII, *Acta Orthop Scand* (1985) **56**: 57–63.
30   Takagi K, Urist MR, The role of bone marrow in bone morphogenic protein induced repair of femoral massive diaphyseal defects, *Clin Orthop* (1982) **171**: 224–31.
31   Urist MR, Leitze A, Mizutani H et al, A bovine low molecular weight bone morphogenic protein (BMP) fraction, *Clin Orthop* (1982) **162**: 219–32.
32   Gray JC, Elves MW, Osteogenesis in bone graft after short term storage and topical antibiotic treatment. An experimental study in rats, *J Bone Joint Surg* (1981) **63B**: 441–5.
33   Clement DA, Papagiannoupoulos G, A complication of the use of suction drains following the removal of intramedullary nails, *J R Coll Surg Edinb* (1987) **32**: 317–318.
34   Blakemore ME, Fractures at cancellous bone graft donor sites, *Injury* (1983) **14**: 519–22.
35   Ubhi CS, Morris DLM, Fracture and herniation of bowel at bone graft donor site in the iliac crest, *Injury* (1984) **16**: 202–203.
36   Mubarak SJ, Carroll NC, Volkmann's contracture in children: aetiology and prevention, *J Bone Joint Surg* (1979) **61B**: 285–93.
37   Müller ME, Allgower M, Schneider R, *Manual of internal fixation* (Springer: Berlin, Heidelberg, New York, 1979).

Chapter 6

1   Allgower M, Border JR, Advances in the care of the multiple trauma patient, *World J Surg* (1983) **7**: 1–3.

2 Orr HW, Compound fractures with special reference to the lower extremity, *Am J Surg* (1939) **46**: 733–7.

3 Trueta J, War surgery of extremities: treatment of war wounds and fractures, *Brit Med J* (1942) **1**: 616–17.

4 Groeningen GK, *Uber den Schock* (JF Bergmann: Wiesbaden, 1885).

5 Erdmann W, Frey R, Madjidi A et al, Oxygen carrying versus non-oxygen carrying colloidal blood substitutes in shock, *Injury* (1982) **14**: 70–4.

6 Jupiter J, Polytrauma, *Seminars in Orthopaedics* (1986) **1**: 201–16.

7 Claudi BF, Meyers NH, Priorities in the treatment of the multiply injured patient with musculoskeletal injuries, in: Meyer MH (Ed) *The mutiply injured patient with complex fractures* (Lea and Febiger: Philadelphia, 1984) 3–9.

8 Wolff, G, Dittman M, Ruedi T et al, Koordination von Chirurgie und Intensivmedizin zur Vermeidung der posttraumatischen respiratorischen Insuffizienz, *Unfallheilkunde* (1978) **81**: 425–42.

9 Messmer KFW, Traumatic shock in polytrauma: Circulatory parameters, biochemistry and resuscitation, *World J Surg* (1983) **7**: 26–30.

10 Gaffney FA, Thal ER, Taylor WF et al, Haemodynamic effects of medical antishock trousers (MAST garment), *J Trauma* (1981) **21**: 931–7.

11 Allgower, M, Burri, C, *Shockindex DMW* (1967) **92**: 1947.

12 Berk, JL, Monitoring the patient in shock. What, when and how? *Surg Clin North Am* (1975) **55**: 713–20.

13 Kreis DJ, Plasencia G, Augenstein D et al, Preventable trauma deaths: Dade County, Florida, *J Trauma* (1986) **26**: 649–52.

14 Burchard KW, Slotman GJ, Jed E et al, Positive pressure respirations and pneumatic antishock garment application—haemodynamic response, *J Trauma* (1985) **25**: 83–9.

15 Committee on Medical Aspects of Automotive Safety: Rating the severity of soft tissue damage. I. The Abbreviated Scale, *JAMA* (1971) **215**: 277–80.

16 Committee on Medical Aspects of Automotive Safety: Rating the severity of soft tissue damage. II. The Comprehensive Scale, *JAMA* (1972) **220**: 717–20.

17 Baker SP, O'Neill B, Haddon W Jr, The injury severity score: A method for describing patients with multiple injuries and evaluating emergency care, *J Trauma* (1974) **14**: 187–96.

18 Goris RJA, Gimbrere JSF, Van Niekerk JL et al, Improved survival of multiply injured patients by early internal fixation and prophylactic mechanical ventilation, *Injury* (1983) **14**: 39–43.

19 Bull JP, Measures of severity of injury, *Injury* (1977) **9**: 184–7.

20 Kirkpatrick JR, Youmans RL, Trauma index: an aide in the evaluation of trauma victims, *J Trauma* (1971) **2**: 711–16.

21 Champion HR, Sacco WJ, Hunt TK. Trauma severity scoring to predict mortality, *World J Surg* (1983) **7**: 4–11.

22 Gormican SP, CRAMS scale: Field triage of trauma victims, *Ann Emerg Med* (1982) **11**: 132–5.

23 Clemmer TP, Orme JF, Thomas F et al, Prospective evaluation of the CRAMS scale for triaging major trauma, *J Trauma* (1985) **25**: 188–91.

24 Gerritsen SM, Van Loenhout T, Gimbrere JSF, Symposium paper: Prognostic signs and mortality in multiply injured patients, *Injury* (1982) **14**: 89–92.

25 Teasdale G, Jennet B, Assessment of coma and impaired consciousness. A practical scale, *Lancet* (1974) **ii**: 81–4.

26 Jennet B, Teasdale G, Galbraith S et al, Severe head injuries in three countries, *J Neurol Neurosurg Psychiat* (1977) **40**: 291–8.

27 Kingma LM, Symposium paper: Radiological management of the patient with multiple injuries, *Injury* (1982) **14**: 17–21.

28 Heiden JS et al, Severe head injury and outcome: a prospective study, in: Popp (Ed), *Neurological trauma* (Raven: New York, 1977).

29 Garland DE, Waters RC, Extremity fractures in head injured adults, in: Meyers MH (Ed), op cit, 134–56.

30 Braakman R, Symposium paper. Emergency craniotomy in severe head injury and the present state of knowledge regarding prognosis, *Injury* (1982) **14**: 22–5.

31 Hoff J, Spetzler R, Winestock D, Head injury and signs of early tentorial herniation, *Western J Med* (1978) **128**: 112–16.

32 Miller JD, Becker DP, Ward JD et al, Significance of intracranial hypertension in severe head injury, *J Neurosurg* (1977) **47**: 503–16.

33 Bakay L, Brain injuries in polytrauma, *World J Surg* (1983) **7**: 42–8.

34 Mattox KL, Thoracic injury requiring surgery, *World J Surg* (1983) **7**: 49–55.

35 Kirsch MM, Management of non-penetrating chest trauma In: Meyers MH (Ed), op cit, 18–32.

36 Kinney JM, Askanazi J, Gump FE et al, Use of ventilatory equivalent to separate hypermetabolism from increased deadspace ventilation in the injured and septic patient, *J Trauma* (1980) **20**: 111–19.

37 Oestern HJ, Sturm JA, Symposium paper: Cardiopulmonary parameters in severe multiple injury, *Injury* (1982) **14**: 75–80.

38 Newman PH, The clinical diagnosis of fat embolism, *J Bone Joint Surg* (1948) **30B**: 290–7.

39 McCarthy B, Mammen E, Leblanc LP et al, Subclinical fat embolism: A prospective study of fifty patients with extremity fractures, *J Trauma* (1973) **13**: 9–16.

40 Avikainen V, Willman K, Rokkanen P, Stress hormones, lipids and factors of haemostasis in trauma. Patients with and without fat embolism syndrome: A comparative study at least one year after severe trauma, *J Trauma* (1980) **20**: 148–53.

41 Bergentz SE, Wilson IA, Effects of trauma on coagulation and fibrinolysis in dogs, *Acta Chir Scand* (1961) **122**: 21–9.

42 Sturm JA, Lewis FR, Trentz O, Cardiopulmonary parameters and prognosis after severe multiple trauma, *J Trauma* (1979) **19**: 305–18.

43 Law DE, Law JK, Brennan R et al, Trauma operating room in conjunction with an air ambulance system: indications, interventions and outcomes, *J Trauma* (1982) **22**: 759–65.

44 Hasset J, Border JR, The metabolic response to trauma and sepsis, *World J Surg* (1983) **7**: 125–31.

45 Schmitz JE, Ahnefeld FW, Burri C, Nutritional support of the multiply injured patient, *World J Surg* (1983) **7**: 132–42.

46   Gann DS, Lilly MP, The neuroendocrine response to multiple trauma, *World J Surg* (1983) **7**: 101–18.

47   MacNicol MF, Prosser AJ, Pulmonary insufficiency after long bone fractures: significant correlation with the catabolic response, *Injury* (1987) **18**: 105–10.

48   Oppenheim WL, Williamson DH, Smith R, Early biochemical changes and severity of injury in man, *J Trauma* (1980) **20**: 135–40.

49   Weil MH, Afifi AA, Experimental and clinical studies on lactate and pyruvate as indicators of the severity of acute circulatory failure (shock), *Circulation* (1970) **XLI**: 989–1001.

50   Booji LHDJ, Symposium paper: Pitfalls in anaesthesia for multiply injured patients, *Injury* (1982) **14**: 81–8.

51   Fairclough JA, Mintowt-Czyz WJ, Mechic I et al, Abdominal girth: An unreliable measure of intra-abdominal bleeding, *Injury* (1984) **16**: 85–7.

52   Goris JA, Draaisma J, Death after blunt injury, *Injury* (1983) **14**: 7–11.

53   Polk HC, Flint LM, Intra-abdominal injuries in polytrauma, *World J Surg* (1983) **7**: 56–67.

54   Heberer G, Becker HM, Dittmer H et al, Vascular injuries in polytrauma, *World J Surg* (1983) **7**: 68–79.

55   Sibbet RR, Palmaz JC, Garina F et al, Trauma of the extremities: Prospective comparison of digital and conventional angiography, *Radiology* (1986) **160**: 179–82.

56   Tscherne H, Ostern HJ, Sturm J, Osteosynthesis of major fractures in polytrauma, *World J Surg* (1983) **7**: 80–7.

57   Whitesides TE, Haney TC, Marimoto K et al, Tissue pressure measurements as a determinant for the need of fasciotomy, *Clin Orthop* (1975) **113**: 45–51.

58   Rorabeck CH, The slit catheter—A new device for measuring intra-compartment pressure, *Proceedings of the Canadian Orthopaedic Research Society*, 14th Annual Meeting (Calgary, Canada, 1980) 12.

59   Mubarak SJ, Owen CA, Double incision fasciotomy of the leg for decompression in compartment syndromes, *J Bone Joint Surg* (1977) **59A**: 184–7.

60   Schulze-Bergmann G, Verletzungen der Arteria poplitea, *Chirurg* (1974) **45**: 391.

61   Nunley JA, Koman A, Urbaniak JR, Arterial shunting as an adjunct to major limb revascularisation, *Ann Surg* (1981) **193**: 271–3.

62   Hasset J, Cerra FB, Siegel J et al, Symposium paper: Multiple systems organ failure—a very brief summary, *Injury* (1982) **14**: 93–7.

63   Gustilo RB, Mendoza RM, Williams DN, Problems in management of Type III (severe) open fractures: A new classification of Type III open fractures, *J Trauma* (1984) **24**: 742–6.

64   Tscherne H, The management of open fractures, in: Tscherne H, Gotzen L (Eds), *Fractures with soft tissue injuries* (Springer: New York, 1984) 10–32.

65   Patzakis MJ, Harvey JP, Ilver D, The role of antibiotics in the management of open fractures, *J Bone Joint Surg* (1974) **56A**: 532–41.

66   Seibel R, Laduca J, Hasset JM et al, Blunt multiple trauma (ISS 36). Femur traction and the pulmonary septic state, *Ann Surg* (1985) **202**: 283–95.

67   Johnson KD, Cadambi A, Burton Seibert G, Incidence of adult respiratory distress syndrome in patients with multiple musculoskeletal injuries. Effect of early operative stabilisation of fractures, *J Trauma* (1985) **25**: 375–7.

68   Goris RJA, The injury severity score, *World J Surg* (1983) **7**: 12–18.

69   Meek RN, Vivoda EE, Pirani S, Comparison of mortality of patients with multiple injuries according to type of fracture treatment—a retrospective age and injury matched series, *Injury* (1986) **17**: 2–4.

70   Riska EB, Myllynen P, Fat embolism in patients with multiple injuries, *J Trauma* (1982) **22**: 891–4.

71   Ruedi T, Wolff G, Vermeidung posttraumatischer Komplikationen durch fruhe definitive Versorgung von Polytraumatiserien mit Frakturen des Bewengsapparats, *Helv Chir Acta* (1975) **42**: 507–12.

72   Lindsey D, Teaching the initial management of major multiple system trauma, *J Trauma* (1980) **20**: 160–2.

Chapter 7

1   Lewinnek GE, Kelsey J, White AA III et al, The significance and a comparative analysis of the epidemiology of hip fractures, *Clin Orthop* (1980) **152**: 35–43.

2   Aaron JE, Gallagher JC, Nordin BEC, Seasonal variation of histological osteomalacia in femoral neck fractures, *Lancet* (1974) **ii**: 84–5.

3   Wilton TJ, Hosking DJ, Pawley E et al, Screening for osteomalacia in elderly patients with femoral neck fractures, *J Bone Joint Surg* (1987) **69B**: 765–9.

4   Lindahl O, Mechanical properties of dried defatted spongy bone, *Acta Orthop Scand* (1976) **47**: 11–19.

5   Newton-John HF and Morgan DB, The loss of bone with age, osteoporosis, and fractures, *Clin Orth Rel Res* (1970) **71**: 229–52.

6   Mazess RB, On aging bone loss, *Clin Orthop* (1982) **165**: 239–52.

7   Riggs BL, Wahner HW, Seeman E et al, Changes in bone mineral density of the proximal femur and spine with aging—differences between the post menopausal and senile osteoporosis syndromes, *J Clin Invest* (1982) **70**: 716–23.

8   Matkovic V, Kostial K, Simonivic I et al, Bone status and fracture rates in two regions of Yugoslavia, *Am. J. Clin Nutr* (1979) **32**: 540–9.

9   Nordin BEC, Need AG, Morris HA et al, New approaches to the problems of osteoporosis, *Clin Orthop Rel Res* (1985) **200**: 181–97.

10   Cummings SR, Are patients with hip fractures more osteoporotic? *Am J Med* (1983) **78**: 487–94.

11   Wasnich RD, Ross PD, Heilbrun LK et al, Prediction of postmenopausal fracture risk with use of bone mineral measurements, *Am J Obstet Gynecol* (1985) **153**: 745–51.

12   Speed K, The unsolved fracture, *Surg Gynec Obstet* (1935) **60**: 341–52.

13   Phemister DB, Fractures of the neck of the femur, *Surg Gynec Obstet* (1934) **59**: 415–40.

14   Smith-Petersen MN, Cave EF, Vangorder GW, Intracapsular fractures of the neck of the femur. Treatment by internal fixation, *Arch Surg* (1931) **23**: 715–59.

15 Goody-Moreira FE, A special stud-bolt screw for fixation of fractures of the neck of the femur, *J Bone Joint Surg* (1940) **38**: 683–7.

16 Pugh WC, A self adjusting nail-plate for fractures about the hip joint, *J Bone Joint Surg* (1955) **37A** 1085–93.

17 Barnes R, Brown JT, Garden RS et al, Subcapital fractures of the femur, *J Bone Joint Surg* (1976) **58B**: 2–24.

18 Moore AT, The self-locking metal hip prosthesis, *J Bone Joint Surg* (1957) **39A**: 811–27.

19 Maxted MJ, Denham RA, Failure of hemiarthroplasty for fractures of the neck of the femur, *Injury* (1984) **15**: 224–6.

20 Sim FM, Staubber RN, Management of hip fractures by total hip arthroplasty, *Clin Orthop* (1980) **152**: 191–7.

21 Riley TBM, Knobs or screws? A prospective trial of prosthetic replacement against internal fixation of subcapital fractures, *J Bone Joint Surg* (1978) **60B**: 136.

22 Sikorski JM, Barrington R, 'Internal fixation versus hemiarthroplasty for the displaced subcapital fracture of the femur, *J Bone Joint Surg* (1981) **73B**: 357–61.

23 Soreide O, Molster A, Raugstad TS, Internal fixation versus primary prosthetic replacement in acute femoral neck fractures: A prospective randomised clinical study, *Br J Surg* (1979) **66**: 56–60.

24 Outerbridge RE, Perosseous venography in the diagnosis of viability in subcapital fractures of the femur, *Clin Orthop* (1978) **137**: 132–9.

25 Milligan GF, The use of kitow fast green to measure the viability of the head of the femur after fractures of the neck of the femur, *Injury* (1979) **10**: 235–8.

26 Flynn M, A new method of reduction of fractures of the neck of the femur based on anatomical studies of the hip, *Injury* (1974) **5**: 309–17.

27 Bentley G, Impacted fractures of the neck of the femur, *J Bone Joint Surg* (1968) **50B**: 551–61.

28 Evans EM, Treatment of trochanteric fractures of the femur, *J Bone Joint Surg* (1949) **31B**: 190–203.

29 Holt EP, Hip fractures in the trochanteric region: treatment with a strong nail and early weight bearing. A report of 100 cases, *J Bone Joint Surg* (1963) **45A**: 687–705.

30 Sarmiento A, Williams EM, The unstable intertrochanteric fracture treatment with a valgus osteotomy and I beam nail-plate. A preliminary report of 100 cases, *J Bone Joint Surg* (1970) **52A**: 1309–18.

31 Mulholland RC, Gunn DE, Sliding screw plate fixation of intertrochanteric femoral fractures, *J Trauma* (1972) **12:7**: 581–91.

32 Dimon JH, Hughston JC, Unstable intertrochanteric fractures of the hip, *J Bone Joint Surg* (1967) **49A:3**: 440–50.

33 Hunter G, Krajbich I, Results of medial displacement osteotomy for unstable intertrochanteric fractures of the femur, *J Bone Joint Surg* (1979) **61B**: 248.

34 Marsh CH, Use of Enders nails in unstable trochanteric femoral fractures, *J Roy Soc Med* (1983) **74**: 550–4.

35 McQuillan W. M., Abernathy PJ, Guy JG, Subcapital fractures of the neck of the femur treated by double-divergent fixation, *Brit J Surg* (1973) **60XI**: 859–66.

36 Jensen JS, Tondevold E, Sorensen P, Long term mortality from femoral neck fracture, *Injury* (1979) **10**: 289–96.

37 Blessed G, Tomlinson BE, Roth M, The association between quantitative measures of dementia and of senile change in the cerebral matter of elderly subjects, *Br J Psychiatry* (1968) **114**: 797–811.

38 Kenzora JE, McCarthy RE, Lowell JD et al, Hip fracture mortality, *Clin Orthop* (1984) **186**: 45–56.

39 Ceder L, Thorngren KG, Wallden B, Prognostic indicators and early home rehabilitation in elderly patients with hip fractures, *Clin Orthop* (1980) **152:** 173–84.

40 Boyd RU, Hawthorne J, Wallace WA et al, The Nottingham Orthogeriatric Unit after 100 admissions, *Injury* (1983) **15**: 193–6.

41 Jensen GF, Christiansen C, Boesen J et al, Epidemiology of postmenopausal spinal and long bone fractures: a unifying approach to postmenopausal osteoporosis, *Clin Orthop* (1982) **166**: 75–81.

42 Hutchinson TA, Polansky SM, Feinstein AR, Postmenopausal oestrogens protect against fractures of hip and distal radius: a case control study, *Lancet* (1979) **ii**: 705–709.

43 Parfitt AM, Dietary risk factors for age-related bone loss and fractures, *Lancet* (1983) **ii**: 1181–4.

44 Horsman A, Gallagher JC, Simpson M et al, Prospective trial of oestrogen and calcium in postmenopausal women, *Br Med J* (1977) **2**: 789–92.

45 Recker RR, Saville PD, Heaney RP, Effect of oestrogens and calcium carbonate on bone less in postmenopausal women, *Ann Intern Med* (1977) **87**: 649–55.

46 Nilas I, Christiansen C, Rodbro P, Calcium supplementation and postmenopausal bone loss, *Br Med J* (1984) **289**: 1103–1106.

47 Consensus Conference: Osteoporsis, *JAMA* (1984) **252**: 799–802.

48 Weiss NS, Ure CL, Ballard JH et al, Decreased risk of fractures of the hip and lower forearm with postmenopausal use of oestrogens, *N Engl J Med* (1980) **303**: 1195–8.

49 Antunes CMF, Stolley PD, Rosenshein NB et al, Endometrial cancer and oestrogen use, *N Engl J Med* (1979) **300**: 9–13.

50 Whitehead MI, Townshend PT, Pryse-Davies J et al, Effects of various types and dosages of progestogens on the postmenopausal endometrium, *J Reprod Med* (1982) **27**: 539–48.

51 Riggs BL, Seeman E, Hodgson SF et al, Effect of fluoride/calcium regimen on vertebral fracture occurrence in postmenopausal osteoporosis, *N Engl J Med* (1982) **306**: 444–50.

52 Kanis JA, Meunier PJ, Should we use fluoride to treat osteoporosis?: A review, *Q J Med* (1984) **210**: 145–64.

Chapter 8

1 Howard, JL, Urist MR, Fracture dislocations of the radius and the ulna at the elbow joint, *Clin Orthop* (1958) **12**: 276–84.

2 Malgaigne JC, Considerations cliniques sur les fractures de la rotule et leur traitement par les griffes, *J Conn Med Prat* (1853) **16**: 9.

3   Firica A, Troianescu O, Fracture comminutive de la tête radiale; technique de reconstruction chiruricale, *Rev Chir Orthop* (1979) **65**: 66–7.

4   Odenheimer K, Harvey JP, Internal fixation of fracture of the head of the radius, *J Bone Joint Surg* (1979) **61A**: 785–7.

5   Herbert TJ, Fisher WE, Management of the fractured scaphoid using a new bone screw, *J Bone Joint Surg* (1984) **66B**: 114–23.

6   Bunker TD, Newman JH, The Herbert differential pitch screw in displaced radial head fractures, *Injury* (1985) **16**: 621–4.

7   Bunker TD, Scott TD, MacNamee PB, A multicentre study of the Herbert differential pitch bone screw for scaphoid fractures, *J Bone Joint Surg* (1987) **69B**: 631–8.

8   MacNamee PB, Bunker TD, Scott TD, The Herbert differential pitch bone screw for articular and osteochondral fractures, *J Bone Joint Surg* (1988) **70B**: 145–6.

9   Benninghoff A, Form und Ban der Gelenkknopel in ihren Bezeihungen zur Funktion, *Zeitschrift fur Zellforschung und Mikroskopien Anatomie* (1925) **2**: 783–862.

10 MacConnail MA, The movement of bones and joints 4; The mechanical structure of articular cartilage. *J Bone Joint Surg* (1951) **33B**: 251–7.

11 Broom ND, Further insight into the structural principles governing the function of articular cartilage, *J Anat* (1984) **139**: 275–94.

12 Mankin HJ, Lippiello L, The turnover of adult rabbit articular cartilage, *J Bone Joint Surg* (1969) **51A**: 1591–1600.

13 Thompson RC Jr, Onega TR Jr, Metabolic activity of articular cartilage in osteoarthritis. An in vivo study, *J Bone Joint Surg* (1979) **61A**: 407–16.

14 Sevitt S, *Bone repair and fracture healing in man* (Churchill Livingstone, Edinburgh, London, New York, 1981).

15 Lane JM, Brighton CT, Menkowitz BJ, Anaerobic and aerobic metabolism in articular cartilage, *J Rheumatol* (1977) **4**: 334–42.

16 Schwartz ER, Kirkpatrick PR, Thompson RC, The effect of environment pH on glycosaminoglycan metabolism by normal chondrocytes, *J Lab Clin Med* (1976) **87**: 198–205.

17 Paloski, MH, Brandt KD, Effect of calcipenia on proteoglycan metabolism and aggregation in normal articular cartilage in vivo, *Biochem J* (1979) **182**: 399–406.

18 Mankin HJ, Conger KA, The acute effects of intraarticular hydrocortisone on articular cartilage in rabbits, *J Bone Joint Surg* (1966) **48AII**: 1383–8.

19 Repo RU, Finlay JB, Survival of articular cartilage after controlled impact, *J Bone Joint Surg* (1977) **59A**: 1068–76.

20 Meachim G, The effects of scarification on articular cartilage of the rabbit, *J Bone Joint Surg* (1963) **45B**: 150–61.

21 Thompson RC Jr, An experimental study of surface injury to articular cartilage and enzyme responses within the joint, *Clin Orthop* (1975) **107**: 239–48.

22 Ghadially FN, Thomas I, Oryschak AF, La Ronde JM, Long-term results of superficial defects in articular cartilage. A scanning electron microscope study, *J Pathol* (1977) **121**: 213–17.

23 De Palma AF, McKeever CD, Subin SK, Process of repair of articular cartilage demonstrated by histology and autoradiology with tritiated thymidine, *Clin Orthop* (1966) **48**: 229–42.

24 Salter RB, Simmonds DF, Malcolm BW et al, The biological effect of continuous passive motion on the healing of full-thickness defects in articular cartilage, *J Bone Joint Surg* (1980) **62A**: 1232–51.

25 Mitchell N, Shephard N, Healing of articular cartilage in intra-articular fractures in the rabbit, *J Bone Joint Surg* (1980) **62A**: 628–34.

26 Faithful DK, Herbert TJ, Small joint fusion of the hand using the Herbert bone screw, *J Hand Surg* (1984) **9B**: 167–8.

27 Russe O, Fracture of the carpal navicular: diagnosis, non-operative treatment and operative treatment, *J Bone Joint Surg* (1960) **42A**: 759–68.

28 Cooney WP, Dobyns JH, Linscheid RL, Fractures of the scaphoid: a rational approach to management, *Clin Orthop* (1980) **149**: 90–7.

29 Stimson LA, Fracture of the carpal scaphoid with dislocation forward of the central fragment, *Ann Surg* (1902) **35**: 574–7.

30 Adams JD and Leonard RD, Fractures of the carpal scaphoid. *New Engl J Med* (1928) **198**: 401.

31 Decoulx P, Rozeman JP, Lemerle P, Les fractures et pseudarthroses du scaphoid carpien, *Lille Chirurgical* (1959) **14**: 113–33.

32 Böhler L, Trojan E, Jahna H, Die Behandlungsergekisse von 734 frischen Bruchen des Kahn bein körpers der Hand, *Wiederherst Traumatol* (1954) **2**: 86.

33 London PS, The broken scaphoid bone: the case against pessimism, *J Bone Joint Surg* (1961) **43B**: 237–44.

34 Leslie IJ, Dickson RA, The fractured carpal scaphoid: natural history and factors influencing outcome, *J Bone Joint Surg* (1981) **63B**: 225–30.

35 Ruby LK Stimson J, Belsky MR, The natural history of scaphoid non-union. A review of fifty-two cases, *J Bone Joint Surg* (1985) **67A**: 428–32.

36 Mack GR, Bosse MJ, Gelberman RH et al, The natural history of scaphoid non-union, *J Bone Joint Surg* (1984) **66A**: 504–509.

37 McLaughlin HL, Parkes JC, Fractures of the carpal navicular (scaphoid) bone; gradations in therapy based on treatment, *J Trauma* (1969) **9**: 311–19.

38 Gasser H, Delayed union and pseudarthrosis of carpal navicular bone: treatment by compression screw osteosynthesis. A preliminary report of 20 fractures, *J Bone Joint Surg* (1965) **47A**: 249–66.

39 Leyshon A, Ireland J, Trickey EL, The treatment of delayed union and non-union of the carpal scaphoid by screw fixation, *J Bone Joint Surg* (1984) **66B**: 124–7.

40 Maudsley RH, Chen SC, Screw fixation in the management of the fractured scaphoid, *J Bone Joint Surg* (1972) **54B**: 432–41.

41 Thomas T, Fractures of the head of the radius, *Univ Penn M Bull* (1905): 184–97.

42 Mason ML, Some observations on fractures of the head of the radius with a review of one hundred cases, *Br J Surg* (1954) **42**: 123–32.

43 Hiem U, Trub HJ, Erfahrungen mit der primaren Osteosynthese von Radiuskopfchonfrakturen, *Helv Chir Acta* (1978) **45**: 63–9.

44 Radin EL, Riseborough J, Fractures of the radial head, *J Bone Joint Surg* (1965) **48AII**: 1055–64.

45 Charnley J, *The closed treatment of common fractures* (E and S Livingstone, Edinburgh, 1950).

46 Adler, JB, Shaftan GW, Radial head fracture: is excision necessary? *J Trauma* (1964) **4**: 115–36.

47 Epstein HC, Wiss DA, Cozen L, Posterior fracture dislocation of the hip with fractures of the femoral head, *Clin Orthop* (1985) **201**: 9–17.

48 Pipkin G, Treatment of grade 4 fracture-dislocation of the hip, *J Bone Joint Surg* (1957) **39A**: 1027–42.

Chapter 9

1 Horak J, Nilsson BE, Epidemiology of fracture of the upper end of the humerus, *Clin Orthop* (1975) **112**: 250–3.

2 Young, TB, Wallace WA, Dunningham T, The long term outcome from fractures of the proximal humerus, in preparation (1988).

3 Neer CS II, Displaced proximal humeral fractures: Part II—Treatment of three-part and four-part displacement, *J Bone Joint Surg (Am)* (1970) **52A**: 1090–1103.

4 Neer CS II, Displaced proximal humeral fractures: Part I—Classification and evaluation, *J Bone Joint Surg* (1970) **52A**: 1077–89.

5 Codman EA, *The shoulder: rupture of the supraspinatus tendon and other lesions in or about the subacromial bursa* (Thomas Todd: Boston, Mass, 1934).

6 Hägg O, Lundberg B, Aspects of prognostic factors in comminuted and dislocated proximal humeral fractures, in: *Surgery of the Shoulder*, Bateman J, Welsh PR (Eds) (BC Decker Inc: Philadelphia, Toronto, 1984) 51–9.

7 Jakob RP, Kristiansen T, Mayo K et al, Classification and aspects of treatment of fractures of the proximal humerus, in: Bateman J, Welsh PR (Eds), op cit, 330–43.

8 Neer CS II, Four-segment classification of displaced proximal fractures, Chapter 9—*Instructional course lectures* (The American Academy of Orthopaedic Surgeons: C.V. Mosby: St Louis, 1975) **XXIV**: 160–8.

9 Wallace WA, Hellier M, Improving radiographs of the injured shoulder, *Radiography* (1983) **49**: 229–33.

10 Clifford PC, Fractures of the neck of the humerus: a review of the late results, *Injury* (1980–81) **12**: 91–5.

11 Lundberg BJ, Svenungson-Hartwig E, Wikmark R, Independent exercises versus physiotherapy in non-displaced proximal humeral fractures, *Scan J Rehab Med* (1979) **11**: 133–6.

12 Young TB, Wallace WA, Conservative treatment of fractures and fracture-dislocations of the upper end of the humerus, *J Bone Joint Surg (Br)* (1985) **67B**: 373–7.

13 Tanner MW, Cofield RH, Prosthetic arthroplasty for fractures and fracture-dislocations of the proximal humerus, *Clin Orthop* (1983) **179**: 116–28.

14 Stableforth PG, Four-part fractures of the neck of the humerus, *J Bone Joint Surg (Br)* (1984) **66B**: 104–8.

15 DePalma AF, Cantilli RA, Fractures of the upper end of the humerus, *Clin Orthop* (1961) **20**: 73–93.

16 Paavolainen P, Björkenheim JM, Slätis P et al, Operative treatment of severe proximal humeral fractures, *Acta Orthop Scand* (1983) **54**: 374–9.

17 Weseley MS, Barenfeld PA, Eisenstein AL, Rush pin intramedullary fixation for fractures of the proximal humerus, *J Trauma* (1977) **17**: 29–37.

18 Rush LV, Rush HC, A technique for longitudinal pin fixation of certain fractures of the ulna and of the femur, *J Bone Joint Surg* (1939) **21**: 619–26.

19 Leyshon RL, Closed treatment of fractures of the proximal humerus, *Acta Orthop Scand* (1984) **55**: 48–51.

20 Neer CS II, Watson KC, Stanton FJ, Recent experience in total shoulder replacement, *J Bone Joint Surg (Am)* (1982) **64A**: 319–37.

21 Redfern TR, Beddow FH, Wallace WA, Clavicular osteotomy in shoulder arthroplasty, in: *The shoulder*, Takagishi N (Ed) (Professional Postgraduate Services: Japan, 1987) 343–5.

22 Kristiansen B, Christensen, SW, Plate fixation of proximal humeral fractures, *Acta Orthop Scand* (1986) **57**: 320–3.

23 Mouradian WH, Displaced proximal humeral fractures—Seven years' experience with a modified Zickel supracondylar device, *Clin Orthop* (1986) **212**: 209–18.

24 Knight RA, Mayne JA, Comminuted fractures and fracture-dislocations involving the articular surface of the humeral head, *J Bone Joint Surg (Am)* (1957) **39A**: 1343–55.

25 DesMarchais JE, Morais G, Treatment of complex fractures of the proximal humerus by Neer hemiarthroplasty, in: Bateman J, Welsh PR (Eds), op cit, 60–2.

26 Kraulis J, Hunter G, The results of prosthetic replacement in fracture-dislocations of the upper end of the humerus, *Injury* (1976) **8**: 129–31.

27 Willems WJ, Lim TE, Neer arthroplasty for humeral fracture, *Acta Orthop Scand* (1985) **56**: 394–5.

28 Hirst P, Wallace WA. Poor results of Neer shoulder replacement in rheumatoid arthritis, in: Takagishi N (Ed), op cit, 362–6.

Chapter 10

1 Hilton J, *On the influence of mechanical and physiological rest in the treatment of accidents and surgical diseases and the diagnostic value of pain* (Bell and Daldy: London, 1863).

2 Thomas HO, *Diseases of the hip, knee and ankle joints with their deformities treated by a new and efficient method* (HK Lewis: London, 1878).

3 Championierre LJ, *Précis du traitement des fractures* (G Steinheil: Paris, 1910).

4 Sarmiento A, A functional below-the-knee cast for tibial fractures, *J Bone Joint Surg* (1967) **49A**: 855–74.

5 Mooney V, Nickel VL, Harvey JP Jr et al, Cast-brace treatment for fractures of the distal part of the femur, *J Bone Joint Surg* (1970) **52A**: 1563–78.

6   Meggitt BF and Thomas TL, A comparative study of methods for treating fractures of the distal half of the femur, *J Bone Joint Surg* (1981) **63B**: 3–6.

7   Wardlaw D, McLaughlan J, Pratt DJ et al, A biomechanical study of cast brace treatment of femoral shaft fractures, *J Bone Joint Surg* (1981) **63B**: 7–11.

8   Sarmiento A, The role of soft tissues in the stabilization of tibial fractures, *Clin Orthop Rel Res* (1974) **105**: 116–29.

9   Sarmiento A, Sobol PA, Sew Hoy AL et al, Prefabricated functional braces for the treatment of fractures of the tibial diaphysis, *J Bone Joint Surg* (1984) **66A**: 1328–39.

10 Roper BA, Functional bracing of femoral fractures, *J Bone Joint Surg* (1981) **63B**: 1–2.

11 Connolly, JF and King P, Closed reduction and early cast-brace ambulation in the treatment of femoral fractures, *J Bone Joint Surg* (1973) **55A**: 1559–80.

12 Sarmiento A, Tarr RR, Sew Hoy AL et al, The evolution and current status of functional fracture bracing, Scientific Exhibit (Booth 8009) 50th annual meeting of the American Academy of Orthopaedic Surgeons, Arnheim, California (1983).

13 Salter R, Simmonds DF, Malcolm BW et al, The biological effects of continuous passive motion on the healing of full thickness defects in articular cartilage, *J Bone Joint Surg* (1980) **62A**: 1238–51.

14 Scotland TR, Wardlaw D, The use of cast-bracing as treatment for fractures of the tibial plateau, *J Bone Joint Surg* (1981) **63B**: 575–8.

15 Beard DJ, Rowley DI, Sharples V et al, Periarticular fractures around the knee joint. The results of 30 cases treated with a femoral cast brace, *J Bone Joint Surg* (1985) **67B**: 145.

16 Mueller ME, Allgower M, Shreider R et al, *Manual of internal fixation* (Springer: Berlin, Heidelberg, New York, 1979).

17 Gill JM, Bowker P, A comparative study of the properties of bandage form splinting materials, *Eng Med* (1982) **11**: 125–34.

18 Rowley DI, Pratt D, Powell ES et al, The comparative properties of Plaster of Paris and Plaster of Paris substitutes, *Arch Orthop Trauma Surg* (1985) **103**: 402–7.

19 Rowley DI, Pratt D, Orthopaedic bandage form splintage materials, *Clinical Materials* (1986) **1**: 1–8.

20 Sarmiento A, Latta LL, *Closed functional treatment of fractures* (Springer: Berlin, Heidelberg, New York, 1985).

21 Duckworth T, *Lecture notes on orthopaedics and fractures* (Blackwell: Oxford, 1980).

22 Kenwright J, Richardson JB, Goodship AE et al, A controlled multicentre study of the influence of axial micromovement on the healing of tibial diaphyseal fractures (BORS, Bradford, 1985: proceedings in print).

23 Kenwright J, Biomechanical measurement of fracture repair, *Biomechanical measurement in orthopaedic practice, Oxford Medical Engineering Series: 5*, Whittle and Harris (Eds) (Clarendon Press: Oxford, 1985).

Chapter 11

1   Maatz R, Lentz W, Arens W et al, *Die Marknagelung und andere intramedulläre Osteosynthesen* (FK Schattauer: Stuttgart, 1983).

2   Senn N, The treatment of fractures of the neck of the femur by immediate reduction and permanent fixation, *JAMA* (1889) 13: 150–9.

3   Lillienthal H, Fracture of the femur: Open operation with introduction of intramedullary splint, *Ann Surg* (1911) **53**: 541–2.

4   Hey Groves EW, Some clinical and experimental observations on the operative treatment of fractures, with especial reference to the use of intramedullary pegs, *Br Med J* (1912) **2**: 1102–5.

5   Hey Groves EW, Treatment of un-united fractures, *Br J Surg* (1918–19) **6**: 203–47.

6   Hey Groves EW, Some contributions to the reconstructive surgery of the hip, *Br J Surg* (1927) Vol XIV, **55**: 486–517.

7   Müller-Meernach, Die Bolzung der Brüche der langen Röhrenknochen, *Zentralbl Chir* (1933) **60**: 1718–23.

8   Küntscher G, *The callus problem* (WH Green: St Louis, 1974) 4.

9   Küntscher G, Die Marknagelung von Knochenbrüchen, *Langenbecks Arch Chir* (1940) **200**: 443–5.

10 Modny MT, Bambara J, The perforated intramedullary nail, *J Am Geriatr Soc* (1953) **1**: 579–88.

11 Kyle RF, Biomechanics of intramedullary nail fixation, *Orthopedics* (1985) **8/11**: 1356–9.

12 Nicod L, Posttraumatische Achsenfehlstellungen an den unteren Extremitäten (Hans Huber: Berne and Stuttgart, 1967).

13 Koostra G, *Femoral shaft fractures in adults* (van Gorcum: Assen, 1973).

14 Müller ME, Posttraumatische Achsenfehlstellungen an den unteren Extremitäten (Hans Huber: Berne and Stuttgart, 1967).

15 Winquist RA, Hansen ST, Clawson DK, Closed intramedullary nailing of femoral fractures, *J Bone Joint Surg* (1984) **66A**: 529–39.

16 Kyle RF, Biomechanics of intramedullary fracture fixation, *Orthopedics* (1985) **8**: 1356–9.

17 Wills R, Turnbaugh T, Brooker AF, Results of preliminary testing of the Brooker Wills nail (Biomet Internal Publication).

18 Papagiannopoulos G, Pratt DJ, Rees PH, Derby intramedullary nail—a biomechanical comparison, *J Biomed Eng* (1985) **7**: 313–17.

19 White GM, Healy WL, Brumback RJ, The treatment of fractures of the femoral shaft with the Brooker Wills distal locking nail, *J Bone Joint Surg* (1986) **68A**: 865–76.

20 Kempf I, Grosse A, Beck G, Closed locked intramedullary nailing, *J Bone Joint Surg* (1985) **67A**: 709–19.

21 Morscher E, Taillard W, *Beinlängenunterscheide* (S Karger: Basle, 1965).

22 Dencker HM, *Fractures of the shaft of the femur* (Orstadius Boktryckerie AB: Göteborg, 1963).

23 Chan KM, Tse PTY, Chow YYN et al, Closed medullary nailing for fractured shaft of the femur, *Injury* (1984) **15**: 381–7.

24 Rokkanen P, Slatis P, Vankka E, Closed or open intramedullary nailing of femoral shaft fractures? *J Bone Joint Surg* (1969) **51B**: 313–23.

25 Smith JEM, The results of early and delayed internal fixation of fractures of the shaft of the femur, *J Bone Joint Surg* (1964) **46B**: 28–31.

26 Charnley J, Guindy A, Delayed operation in the open reduction of the fractures of the long bones, *J Bone Joint Surg* (1961) **43B**: 664–71.

27 Seibel R, Laduca J, Hassett JM et al, Blunt multiple trauma (ISS 36), femur traction, and the pulmonary failure-septic-state, *Ann Surg* (1985) **202**: 283–95.

28 Christie J, Kinninmonth AWG, Court Brown CM et al, The closed interlocking femoral nail; experience and complications in the first 100 patients, *J Bone Joint Surg* (1987) **69BIII**: 489.

29 Seligson D, *Concepts in intramedullary nailing* (Grune and Stratton: New York, 1985).

30 Klemm, in Seligson D, op cit.

31 Papagiannopoulos G, Karpinski MRK, Newton G, Medullary femoral nailing of pathological fractures using the Derby nail—a preliminary report of 22 cases, *Injury* (1986) **17**: 240–7.

32 Rhinelander FW, Circulation of bone, in Bourne GH *The biochemistry and physiology of bone* (Academic Press, London and New York, 1972).

33 Sevitt S, *Bone repair and fracture healing in man* (Churchill Livingstone: Edinburgh, London, New York, 1981).

34 Danckwart Lillieström G, Lorenzi GL, Olerud S, Intramedullary nailing after reaming *Acta Orthop Scand* (1970) Suppl no 134.

35 Yamagishi M, Yoshimura Y, The biomechanics of fracture healing, *J Bone Joint Surg* (1955) **37A**: 1035–68.

36 Panjabi MM, White AA, Wolf JW, A biomechanical comparison of the effects of constant and cyclical compression on fracture healing in rabbit long bones *Acta Orthop Scand* (1979) **50**: 653–61.

37 Goodship A, Kenwright J, The influence of induced micromovement upon the healing of experimental tibial fractures, *J Bone Joint Surg* (1985) **67B**: 650–5.

38 Thomas TL, Meggit BF, A comparative study of methods for treating fractures of the distal half of the femur, *J Bone Joint Surg* (1981) **63B**: 3–6.

Chapter 12

1 Berenger-Feraud LJB, De L'emploi de la pointe de Malgaine dans les fractures, *Rev Ther Med Chir* (1867) **15**: 228, 9–12.

2 Malgaigne JC, Considérations cliniques sur les fractures de la rotule et leur traitement par les griffes, *J Conn Med Prat* (1853) **16**: 9–12.

3 Parkhill C, A new apparatus for the fixation of bone after resection and in fractures with tendency to displacement, *Trans Am Surg Assoc* (1897) **15**: 351–6.

4 Lambotte A, *Chirurgie Operatoire des Fractures* (Masson: Paris, 1913).

5 Hey Groves EW, *On modern methods of treating fractures* (John Wright: Bristol, 1916).

6 Crile DW, Fracture of the femur: A method of holding the fragments in difficult cases, *Br J Surg* (1918) **23**: 458–62.

7 Anderson R, An automatic method of treatment for fractures of the tibia and fibula, *Surg Gynecol Obstet* (1934) **58**: 637–8.

8 Stader O, A preliminary announcement of a new method of treating fractures, *North Am Vet* (1937) **18**: 37.

9 Lewis KM, Breidenbach L, Stader O, The Stader reduction splint for treating fractures of the shafts of the long bones, *Ann Surg* (1942) **116**: 623.

10 Hoffman R, Rotules à os pour la réduction dirigée, non saglante des fractures (Osteotaxis), *Helv Med Acta* (1938) **5**: 844–50.

11 Charnley J, Positive pressure in arthrodesis of the knee joint, *J Bone Joint Surg* (1948) **30B**: 478–80.

12 Judet R, Judet T, Compression dans le traitement des pseudarthrosis. Résultats et techniques, *Mem Acad Chir* (Paris) (1959) **85**: 511.

13 Vidal J, Baumel H, Konirsch G, et al, A propos de la synthese des fractures et pseudarthrosis de l'éxtremité inférieur du femur, *Lyon Chirurgical* (1960) **56**: no 4, 538–45.

14 Burny F, Elastic external fixation of tibial fractures. Study of 1421 cases, in: Brooker AF and Edwards CC, *External fixation, the current state of the art* (Williams and Wilkins: Baltimore, 1979).

15 Ilisarov L, Results of clinical tests and experience obtained from the clinical use of the set of Ilisorov compression—distraction apparatus, *Med Export* (Moscow) (1976) **13**.

16 Volkov MV, Oganesion OV, Restoration of function in the knee and the elbow with a hinged distractor apparatus, *J Bone Joint Surg* (1975) **57A**: 591–600.

17 Green SA, Complications of external skeletal fixation, *Clin Orthop* (1983) **180**: 109–16.

18 Gie GA, MacEachern AG, Experience with the Orthofix: Recent Advances in External Fixation, Riva del Garda (1986).

19 Green SA, *Complications of external fixation. Causes, prevention and treatment* (Thomas, Springfield: Illinois, 1981).

20 Matthews L, Hirsch C, Temperatures measured in human cortical bone when drilling, *J Bone Joint Surg* (1972) **54A**: 297.

21 Mears D, The use of external fixation in arthrodesis, in: Brooker, AF and Edwards CC, op cit.

22 Chao EYS, Pope MH, The mechanical basis of external fixation, in: *Concepts in external fixation*, Seligson D and Pope MH (Eds) (Grune and Stratton: New York, 1982).

23 McKibbin B, Fracture healing, *Surg* (1986) **1**: 796–802.

24 Perren SM, Physical and biological aspects of fracture healing with special reference to internal fixation, *Clin Orthop* (1979) **138**: 175–96.

25 Gentile G, Variodyne method for external osteosynthesis: Recent Advances in External Fixation, Riva del Garda (1986).

26 Yamagishi M, Yoshimura Y, The biomechanics of fracture healing, *J Bone Joint Surg* (1955) **37A**: 1035–68.

27 Goodship A, Kenwright J, The influence of induced

micromovement upon the healing of experimental tibial fractures, *J Bone Joint Surg* (1985) **67B**: 650–5.

28 De Bastiani G, Aldegheri R, Renzi Brivio L, Dynamic axial fixation. A rational alternative for the external fixation of fractures, *Int Orthop* (1986) **10**: 95.

29 McKibbin B, The use of semi-rigid carbon fibre reinforced plastic plates for the fixation of human fractures, *J Bone Joint Surg* (1982) **64B**: 105–11.

30 McKibbin B, Factors affecting the formation of external callus: Recent advances in External Fixation, Riva del Garda (1986).

31 Pringle RM, Dynamic axial fixation—A Scottish experience: Recent Advances in External Fixation, Riva del Garda (1986).

32 Mears DC, *External skeletal fixation* (Williams and Wilkins: Baltimore, 1983), 93–160.

33 Vidal J, Buscayret C, Connes H et al, Open fractures and infected pseudarthroses, *Clin Orthop* (1983) **180**: 83–95.

34 Green SA, Zinar D, Chandler R, Problems with combined internal and external fixation for diaphyseal fractures: Recent Advances in External Fixation, Riva del Garda (1986).

35 Darder A, Gomar F, A series of tibial fractures treated conservatively, *Injury* (1976) **6**: 225–35.

36 Sarmiento A, A functional below the knee cast for tibial fractures, *J Bone Joint Surg* (1967) **49AII**: 855–75.

37 Ruedi T, Webb JK, Allgower M, Experience with the dynamic compression plate (DCP) in 418 recent fractures of the tibial shaft, *Injury* (1976) **7**: 252–7.

38 Holzach P, Matter P, The comparison of steel and titanium dynamic compression plates used for internal fixation of 256 fractures of the tibia, *Injury* (1979) **10**: 120–3.

39 Matter P, Rittman WW, The open fracture (Hans Huber: Berne and Stuttgart, 1977).

40 Seligson, D, Matheny L, Tibia terrible—a sixteen week programme for prevention: Recent Advances in External Fixation, Riva del Garda (1986).

41 Larsson K, Van den Linden W, Open tibial shaft fractures, *Clin Orthop* (1983) **180**: 63–7.

42 Van der Linden W, Larsson K, Plate fixation versus conservative treatment of tibial shaft fractures. Randomised trial, *J Bone Joint Surg* (1979) **61A**: 873–8.

43 Karlstrom G, Olerud S, External fixation of severe open tibial fractures with the Hoffman frame, *Clin Orthop* (1983) **180**: 68–77.

44 Fellander M, Treatment of fractures and pseudarthrosis of the long bones by Hoffman's transfixation method, *Acta Orthop Scand* (1963) **33**: 132–50.

45 Coppola AJ, Anzel SH, Use of the Hoffman external fixator in the treatment of femoral fractures, *Clin Orthop* (1983) **180**: 78–82.

46 Brug E, Pennig D, Gähler R et al, Polytrauma und Femurfraktur, *Akt Traumatol* (1988) **18**: 125–8.

47 Agostini S, Leso P, Results of the treatment of pseudarthrosis using the D.A.F.: Recent Advances in External Fixation, Riva del Garda (1986).

48 Seligson D, External fixation of pelvic fractures, in: Seligson D and Pope MH, op cit, 183–202.

49 Tile M, Pennal GF, Pelvic disruption: Principles of management, *Clin Orthop* (1980) **151**: 56–64.

50 Slatis P, Karaharju EO, External fixation of the pelvic girdle with a trapezoidal compression frame, *Injury* (1975) **7**: 53–6.

51 Vidal J, Nakach G, External fixation in the management of severe fractures of the upper limb: Recent Advances in External Fixation, Riva del Garda (1986).

52 Cooney WP III, Current use of external fixation in upper extremity injuries: Recent Advances in External Fixation, Riva del Garda (1986).

53 Lavini F, Mosconi F, Results of treating the upper limbs with the D.A.F.: Recent Advances in External Fixation, Riva del Garda, (1986).

54 Vidal J, Buscayret C, Connes H, Treatment of articular fractures by ligamentotaxis with external fixation, in: Brooker AF and Edwards CC, op cit.

55 Ombredanne L, L'osteosynthese temporaire chez les enfants, *Presse Med* (1929) **37**: 845–8.

56 O'Connor BT, Trend in modern fracture care, Seminar in dynamic axial fixation, Münster (March 1986).

57 Scott Stanwyck T, Seligson D, External fixation in children's fractures: Recent Advances in External Fixation, Riva del Garda (1986).

58 Charnley J, *Compression arthrodesis* (Churchill Livingstone: Edinburgh, London, New York, 1953).

59 Lance EM, Paval A, Fries I et al, Arthrodesis of the ankle joint. A follow up study, *Clin Orthop* (1979) **142**: 146–58.

60 Ratliff AHC, Compression arthrodesis of the ankle, *J Bone Joint Surg* (1959) **41B**: 524–34.

61 Magerl FP, External spinal skeletal fixation: Recent Advances in External Fixation, Riva del Garda (1986).

62 Olerud S, Sjostrom L, Hamberg MD et al, Anterior fusion for chronic lumbar pain, selection and postoperative stabilisation with an external fixator: Recent Advances in External Fixation, Riva del Garda (1986).

63 Rowe NL, Williams JLL, *Maxillo-facial injuries* (Churchill Livingstone: Edinburgh, London, New York, 1985).

64 Turi G, Tomasi PS, Armotti PA et al, The dynamic axial fixator in directional osteotomy of the knee: Recent Advances in External Fixation, Riva del Garda (1986).

65 MacEachern AG, Gie GA, Valgus osteotomy of the upper tibia for osteoarthrosis of the knee: Recent Advances in External Fixation, Riva del Garda (1986).

66 Sportono L, A new method for the correction of femoral-tibial axial deviations: Recent Advances in External Fixation, Riva del Garda (1986).

67 Pope MH, Seligson D, Frymoyer JW, The future of external fixation, in Seligson D and Pope MH, op cit, 309–13.

68 Gallinaro P, Biasibetti A, Demangos J, Treatment of long bone diaphyseal pseudarthrosis by means of external fixation: Recent Advances in External Fixation, Riva del Garda (1986).

69 Gallinaro M, Rossi P, Dettoni A, et al, Open fractures with loss of bone substance and soft tissue: Remarks on compression—distraction osteosynthesis: Recent Advances in External Fixation, Riva del Garda (1986).

Index

Page numbers in *italic* refer to the illustrations